This isn't just another DIET book—in fact, strike that word from your vocabulary! Here is the official book of the YMCA'S Slim Living program. It contains the same wit, wisdom, and inspiration which has worked in hundreds of cities and thousands of lives.

slim living day by day

JoAnn Ploeger

LIVING BOOKS
Tyndale House Publishers, Inc.
Wheaton, Illinois

Library of Congress Catalog Card Number A 842752.
ISBN 0-8423-5913-3, paper. Copyright © 1977 by JoAnn
Ploeger, 3605 Strawberry Lane, Port Huron, Michigan 48060.
All rights reserved. First Living Books Edition, August 1979.
Printed in the United States of America. No part of this
book may be used or reproduced in any manner whatsoever
without permission, except in case of brief quotations embodied
in critical articles or reviews.

dedication

With love
and with gratitude
for your patience
with all my
quirks
. . . to Jack,
the love of my life,
. . . and Judy,
and Jeanne,
and Jack, Jr.
. . . and little Jill
. . . and to Jan.

contents

foreword

"Everybody needs somebody . . . sometime," the lyrics of the song promise. As I ponder my previous years of gaining and losing and binges and dieting, I have to agree. How I detested the loneliness of self-recrimination and the frustration of unshared pride when reaching a goal; so I thought, "Because someone helped me, I'll help you . . . to help yourself."

Identification with something—or someone—seems to relieve that feeling of loneliness. One psychologist I know observed, "No one can lose weight alone. We need the approval and help of another individual." So here is help. Read on . . . one thought at a time . . . day by day.

I'd like to suggest that you skim through the book once, then come back and leisurely read a chapter at a time, day by day, following the homework as you progress. Test each technique and assignment against your present life-style and ideals. Try each one and accept those that can become a natural part of your life without excess strain and pain. Losing weight can be as simple as changing a few lifelong habits. It won't all happen at once, just as you didn't learn to walk the day after you were born. We have to be taught, very carefully taught, to sit, to creep, to stand, to walk, and only then to run . . . at a jogging pace for the rest of our lives.

Since I'm a new golfer, I'll compare these ideas to my first lessons on the links. The pro told me many things and had me try each one . . . grip the club like this, put your feet like that, keep your head down, follow through when you swing, and on and on. But then he told me to concentrate on learning two new ideas at a time! And it worked! Learn each chosen technique well, until it becomes a habit; then go on to another. That's the only way I can help you help yourself.

Read your daily chapter. Try the technique or take the test. If it helps, place a check in the box by that technique for each day you "follow through." Drop the suggestions which are not appropriate to your life-style; but keep, and *practice, practice, practice* those which help you reach your goal.

When you need a helping hand . . . when you need an encouraging word . . . when you know you are one body who needs somebody, I'll be here. All you've got to lose is unattractive pounds. All you've got to gain is a new Slim Life. Smile!

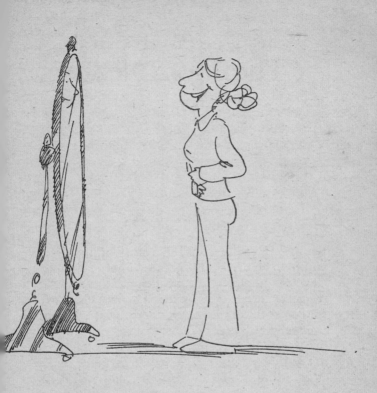

The world is like a mirror
Reflecting what you do.
And if you face it smiling
It will smile right back at YOU.
                              —AUTHOR UNKNOWN

lesson one

Awareness . . .
The Most Necessary
Step

Let me tell you a story . . . a story of life and love and food all blended together. There are no great tragedies in this story, no dramatic events which triggered off a chain of psychotic eating, or resulted in an unattractive body seventy pounds overweight. We all like to feel that we had some deep-seated reason for becoming overweight. Let's not kid ourselves: this is actually true in very few cases. More often, it's a simple matter of drifting into a life-style and not having the knowledge, or the initiative, to pull ourselves back out.

Well, on with our story. Once upon a time a little housewife was madly in love with her husband; she wanted to be the best of everything to him. First, she learned to cook like Mama used to cook . . . not just those everyday things she'd learned as a girl living at home, but to really COOK . . . those yummy pies and cakes to go with staple meat meals. Those would keep a husband happy! Next, she went to her mother-in-law and learned all the recipes that had been HIS childhood favorites; and finally, she pored over cookbooks, magazines, newspapers, and her friends' recipe boxes and came up with a repertoire that was the equal of the finest French chef. This became the goal of her new life ... to take the best of what everyone had to teach and put it together in grand style; because, after all, wasn't the way to a man's heart through his stomach?

Ah, but enter a new dimension into our story ... add three little children, each a year apart, and each demanding equal time. The goal to become the gourmet chef was set aside to allow more time for her to care for new responsibilities; our little housewife began to prepare only the quickest and easiest dishes.

But life goes on, and as everyone knows, little bundles of joy become bigger bundles of concern. When the physical care lessens, the mental care begins. And little Mama solved all her problems with the great pacifier ... the wise sage ... the soothsayer of all times ... FOOD. Every problem, great or small, could be solved by eating. And, not really having any goal, except to get through one day at a time, her life went on. Then one day little Mama woke up, not so little and not so young. Looking back at her in the full-length mirror was a fat, middle-aged lady. And her husband, too, had to admit that he had picked up unattractive excess weight. Was it too late? Is it ever too late? Not at all. Each of us stops to take that look at different stages of our lives. The awareness of the problem and the desire to do something about it are the best motivating forces in the world. Is today your day to awaken? I hope so!

Now that the eyes are open . . . let's take that first step and evaluate what the problem is. And let's begin to do something about it. Below is a little quiz I wish you'd take. Get your pencil out and write on the pages. Then let each member of your family provide his own answers.

EATING BEHAVIOR QUIZ

Check each statement which seems appropriate to your life-style at this time or in the past.

_____ I eat too fast at meals.

_____ I eat between meals at least three times a day.

_____ I eat good-sized portions of meat and bread.

_____ I realize I eat too many sweet and starchy foods.

_____ Though I'm busy, I'm not physically active every day.

_____ I'm certain there is a physical cause for my being overweight.

_____ There are times when I eat because I'm bored or don't want to do some tasks which need doing.

_____ I feel my overweight is "creeping obesity" . . . adding a few pounds each year.

_____ I can't really tell when I'm full or have had enough, so that I can stop eating.

_____ Many times I overeat to take my mind off other problems.

_____ I sometimes "reward" myself for doing a good job or for doing something distasteful to me . . . by eating.

_____ I eat most often when I'm with other people.
___✓___ I overeat usually when I'm alone.
_____ I very often grab stand-up snacks.
___✓___ I always finish the food on my plate.
_____ I stop eating when I feel full.
_____ I stop eating when everyone else is finished, even though I'd like to have a little more of some things.
_____ I stop eating when I feel satisfied.

Now total your answers. If you have more than five or six True answers, we can work on your eating behavior. The first step is the *awareness* of your eating habits. Next, take steps toward changing those habits inappropriate to your goal.

One technique stands out above all others in learning to control your weight. *Keep a food intake diary* ... every day ... for the rest of your life, or for as long as you need to, until you feel really comfortable with food control ... until *you* are master of the situation. An example is given in Figure 1. Make this your model for life. Each week keep your weekly food intake sheet. Each time you eat something, write it down immediately; don't wait until evening and put it all down at one time. (It's too easy to forget some foods, even though your body doesn't forget to add them.) Then, at the end of each day, go back and reevaluate. Put a line under the foods which you might have omitted or changed, those foods which keep you from your determined goal. No recriminations are necessary; just be realistic about what happened. We'll take the next step tomorrow.

Technique for the day: Keep a food inventory list ... every day (see Figure 1). Each time you do,

15

give yourself a check in the box for the day (see page 146).

> *Just for today . . . I will try to live through this day only,*
> *And not tackle my whole life problem at once.*
> *I can do something for twelve hours that would appall me if I felt I had to keep it up for a lifetime.*

—KENNETH HOLMES

FIGURE 1.

FOOD INTAKE INVENTORY FORM　　　　DAY　　　　NAME

FOOD: AMOUNT	FOOD INVENTORY LIST	TIME OF DAY AND LENGTH OF TIME	SOCIAL DEGREE OF HUNGER (0-4)		PLACE: HOME, WORK RESTAURANT RECREATION	MOOD: ANXIOUS BORED TIRED DEPRESSED ANGRY HAPPY	1. OTHER ACTIVITY 2. BODY POSITION
			ALONE	WITH:			

17

lesson two

Be Realistic
in Setting Goals

Good morning! Or is it afternoon or evening before you've found a chance to sit down and read your Slim Living daily encouragement? Before you get too comfortable in the easy chair, run quickly and find your driver's license.

All set? Does it have your weight listed on it? I understand some states no longer require this since so many people stretch the truth (toward the lower end of the scale, of course). If you do have weight listed on yours, how truthful is it? Less than you actually weighed at that time? Or have you lost some weight since you secured that last license?

Now take a look inside your billfold. Do you have a picture of yourself? How about of other people ... whose picture do you have in there? Why not one of yourself?

All of these little tests point up the fact that we

aren't always as honest with ourselves or others as we'd like to think we are. We mentally picture ourselves a bit thinner than we actually are. One lady told me the smartest thing she ever did was invest in four full-length mirrors, which she placed strategically around her home. You can't hide from the truth when it faces you at each corner.

Today is the day to take a good look at ourselves and make a decision. Once we've decided it really is time to get down to basic good food—and once we've decided on a sensible plan, not one of those three-week wonders—we need to take a long-range look and determine exactly how much weight we should lose and how quickly we should lose it. The first question most people ask is, "How much can I lose in a month?" To be truthful, there is no standard answer to that question.

Scientists tell us we are capable of losing about 1 percent of our body weight per week, averaged out over a period of time. What does that mean for you? If you are 175 pounds, it might mean about 1½ to 1¾ pounds per week. Granted, every week won't be the same. Some will be most encouraging and others, even when you feel you have been especially diligent, will be disappointing.

Mathematically, an average woman twenty-four to forty-five years old burns about 1,600 calories per day, unless she is excessively active. A man burns about 2,000. We must burn 3,500 calories to lose one pound. Put this on paper for yourself . . . if we use 1,600 calories per day, and need 500 less than that per day to lose one pound a week, that means we must eat 500 calories less than the 1,600 per day or burn 500 calories more per day by movement and exercise. Most nutritionists agree that the average woman should not go below the 1,200 calorie intake per day, and most men should consume at least 1,600 calories per day to be well-nourished. Now, *you* determine what is a good weight for you. Determine how many calories you should consume daily, how fast you might plan to lose weight sensibly. Put your projected losses on the graph in Figure 2. Weigh yourself each week and follow the graph in a different color of ink to check your progress.

Assignment for the day: Set your goals realistically. Weigh yourself and begin your weekly weight graph. Each week that you weigh and fill in your graph, give yourself a check in the box for the day. Be patient, conscientious, and consistent. As the graph turns downward, your pride in accomplishment will turn upward. It's the beginning of a new you. Congratulations!

> *The measure of success is not whether you have a tough problem to deal with, but whether it's the same problem you had last year.*
> —JOHN FOSTER DULLES

FIGURE 2.

Weight

Begin . . . ───────────

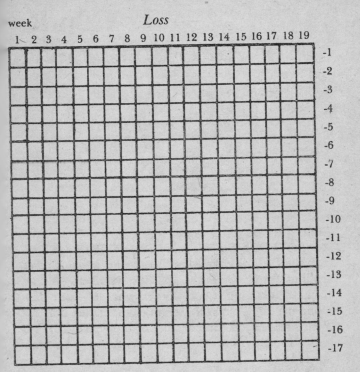

week   *Loss*

1 2 3 4 5 6 7 8 9 10 11 12 13 14 15 16 17 18 19

lesson three

The Pride
of Accomplishment

Well, did you do it again? Are you a "four-day wonder"? Or have you gone beyond that stage and into the fifth day, or even the second week of controlling foods? Are you patting yourself on the back? ... Or don't you know what a "four-day wonder" is? That's someone who makes a New Year's resolution (on any day of the year) to go on a diet and then four days later *wonders* why he ever started.

Physicians tell us that most "diets" last from four days to two weeks. You realize when you say "I'm going ON a diet" that you can "go off" it as well.

Diets have the highest incidence of failure of anything we attempt. Only 20 percent of the people who begin a diet ever lose ten to forty pounds and keep them off for a year's time. If I could, I would eliminate the word "diet" from the English language. It's a failure word from the beginning. In our minds we say, "I've tried this before and failed, and I probably won't make it this time either." It's a negative, self-defeating word. Let's strike it from our personal vocabularies. That's our introduction to a new Slim Life. Never again will we say D-I-E-T; rather, say: "This is my way of life."

Imagine it now . . . we're at a party and someone smirks, "You're not eating a thing! Are you on a diet again?" With a smile on our face we answer, "No, I'm living." And we can mean it. Being aware of what's going on around us, seeing everything clearly with eyes open, can be living in a way we never lived before.

Or . . . Mother says, "Have some of my pecan pie, Honey, I made it just for you." We answer gently, "Mom, pecan pie isn't in my life." Did you note the difference: We didn't complain, "It's not on my diet." We avoided that negative word again . . . and answered, "It's not in my life."

Now, the word "life" is happy; I'm certainly happy that I'm living! Each day is exciting and challenging. How dull, how boring it would be if we allowed life to be humdrum, routine, the same old thing each day. Living life to the fullest means some determination, some really hard work . . . but loads of fun when you and I accomplish a goal that we know took "hard work."

How good it feels to look at a clean kitchen floor that we have just scrubbed on hands and knees. How marvelous to hug a little child with dry panties when it has taken weeks and even months to train that child. What a thrill to try on a dress that we've just stitched up on the old sewing ma-

chine. We're proud of each accomplishment. . . .
And yet, each task required hard work and determination. We took just one step at a time. The little
one wasn't trained by saying, "Abracadabra" . . .
Oh, no! And the sewing doesn't always come out
right the very first time; it may take some ripping
and repeating before we're satisfied. The scrubbed
floor will become dirty again, but for now, it's
sparkling clean. Each task we've avoided will make
us proud when it's tackled and finished. So, too,
will each step we take along the way in our new
Slim Life.

Just for today, what step will you take that will
give you the pride of accomplishment? Set a daily
goal, then hold your head up and say, "I did it."
Choose a work task for today . . . do it, and give
yourself a check in the box marked *Accomplishment*.
Learn to count every planned and completed event
with pride! See page 146.

lesson four

Motivation

Much material has been written about the behavior of overeating. I use many prevention techniques daily to exist in my Slim Life. Let's look at some of the questions which arise when psychologists explore the minds of overweight Americans, and see what we can discover about ourselves.

Does research prove that human behavior is determined by inherited tendencies or by what people learn? Truthfully, research has not decided just which things determine our behavior, or just how much each thing contributes. There are controversies among professionals regarding what part of our behavior is formulated by daily learning experiences and what part is inherited. Behavioral science is making inroads into this study and will have much to contribute in the future.

What part do individual needs and recognitions

play in the studies of obesity? Experts agree that we, as human beings, have the same basic needs: food, shelter, air, and other biological necessities; safety and security; love, communication with others, and self-esteem—if we are to reach our highest potential. However, these needs will vary in intensity and degree with each of us. We must build a sort of pyramid as we satisfy each need, usually not moving on to another level until the basics are met. For example, we *must* have enough money for food before we move on to the desire to save money. These needs of ours become motivators in our lives. What we often "do" is definitely connected with meeting our needs. We all have the need for recognition, to feel, "I am somebody." In many cases where there is lack in our lives, the lack becomes a motivator for choosing *food* to meet the need.

Being AWARE of these needs is the first step in solving our problem . . . overeating. See how many of these reasons for eating strike a chord in your pattern. I eat because:

It gives me pleasure.

I like the taste.

Everybody's doing it.

It's tradition.

It's expected of me.

Food is readily available.

The doctor told me to.

I must stay alive.

I want to attain a desired weight.

I want good health.

I must maintain my present weight without gaining.

I'm hungry.

It shows success, wealth, and prestige.

I'm frustrated.

I'm depressed.

I'm rewarding myself.

It pleases someone.

I feel lonely, isolated, rejected.

I'm bored, there's nothing else to do.

It's a matter of habit.

It relieves nervous tension.

I can't think of anything but food.

I'm tempted by pictures and recipes in advertising.

It gives me a feeling of strength and power.

How many of these reasons have you and I used in the past? Just today let's begin to open our eyes and our sensitivities to the reasons for eating. They may be perfectly legitimate reasons; we need not think we are committing a crime. Let's open our eyes to awareness.

Assignment: During at least one meal or snack today, analyze your feelings and reasons for eating. Write down the emotion you experience (each in a different colored pen or pencil) on your food inventory sheet. If there is a time when you devour high-calorie foods, try to use that time to analyze your feelings. Be honest with yourself. Each day that you do this, give yourself a check in the box for the day. See page 146.

Dear Lord, I come confessing.
To live dangerously in these days is unavoidable.
But to live ignorantly is inexcusable.
And I live ignorantly.

. . . I don't plan my days. They just come.
I don't plan my tomorrows either.
Mine is a "live one day at a time" casualness
that constitutes living ignorantly.

. . . Lord, God,
I would live intentionally.
Thought-fully,
Not by default,
but by design.
Amen.

—from **BLESS THIS MESS**

lesson five

A Lucky Day

We're always looking for the pot of gold at the end of the rainbow. Is this how we look at losing weight? Do we hop on the scales hoping we have lost five pounds miraculously and overnight? Losing weight is not LUCK. It takes day by day discipline and hard work ... but how rewarded we feel when we accomplish the loss of a pound a week. That adds up to fifty pounds in one year! ... Fifty pounds ... while learning other things about myself so I can live meaningfully. Treating my body like the gift from God that it is! Isn't that much better than luck?

And what joy! A ten-pound loss makes me feel like kicking up my heels and jumping up and down. The accomplishment of a goal can bring untold feelings of pride. Our self-esteem is newly won and music flows from every fiber of our being.

There is no "luck" involved with controlling this lust for foods. Let's set one goal a day for ourselves and meet it.

One goal a day? One goal at a time? That's what we're doing. What's today's idea? Let's concentrate

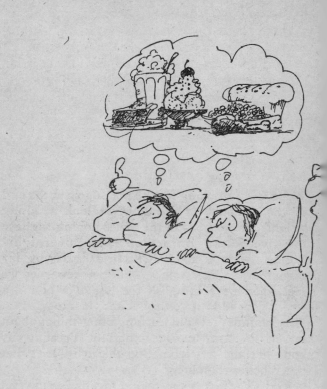

on slowing down and delaying the act of eating. Let's be aware of what we are consuming. Eating slowly usually causes you to eat less and it gives foods a better chance of being absorbed into the system, thus decreasing hunger. If we take at least twenty minutes per meal, we will feel full and satisfied, even though we consume less food.

Today we ask you to concentrate on putting your fork down between bites. You'll eat more slowly. It will take a real awareness since it is far from natural at this point. BEGIN BY LAYING YOUR FORK DOWN BETWEEN EVERY FOUR BITES. Chew and swallow the food before taking another bite. When you find this comfortable, stop once every three bites, then every two bites, until you reach the best ratio ... one to one.

On the record sheet today, begin marking the ratio as you use this technique for each meal. Instead of just marking with the usual X, use ratio figures. For example: 1:4, if you lay your fork down every four bites; 1:3, for every three bites; and so forth, to the ultimate goal of 1:1 ratio. Just try it one meal a day to start and see if you can, over a period of time, make it a regular habit. See how much more satisfied and full you feel after you become accustomed to this technique. It will be frustrating at first, as are all new things which cause us to concentrate ... but I'm willing to bet you find it a most helpful idea. This is a game you play at home, by yourself, and it doesn't cost a penny.

Set your sights high. Shoot for the moon ... when you lose ten pounds, praise the Lord!

Just for today . . . I will have a program.
I may not follow it exactly but I will have it.
I will save myself from two pests—hurry and
*   indecision.*

—KENNETH HOLMES

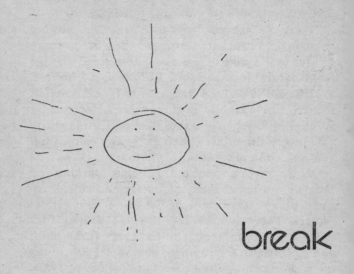

break

It's time for a pause in our reading and working schedule. So far we've concentrated on you and your problem. You like to overeat . . . and so do I. Face it. Admit it. Record it.

Now we're ready to move on, to offer solutions. Forward march, and conquer . . . . . day by day!

lesson six

It Takes Work!

"You can't teach an old dog new tricks!" That sounds like something my grandmother might have said. Most often an adage for any situation is really an excuse for not motivating ourselves for change.

Motivating . . . motivation . . . don't you get tired of that word? Does it make you feel like a failure? Yet, that's what it's all about. To control our weight, we must *motivate* ourselves to change old habits that have not given us the results we desire.

Today, let's talk about another step toward that change. Acceptance . . . acceptance of ourselves as human beings, not perfect, but with faults . . . like everyone else. Accept the fact that we have, unconsciously, developed habits that are not giving us the overall well-being that will keep our bodies in the shape we'd like. Our overeating habits developed over a period of time, so stealthily that we really weren't aware there was a change.

We habitually turn to food to compensate for lack of other satisfactions (lack of love, boredom, anxiety, depression); for needs other than hunger or good nutrition.

Certainly the fact that relatively few overcome and control obesity over a lifetime indicates that the strength of old eating habits and the reality of daily needs are in constant conflict. Although we believe in good nutrition and physical fitness, our emotions, prejudices, taboos, prestige symbols, and other influences often outweigh our knowledge, judgment, and even experience in determining eating habits.

You and I must *accept* the fact that the "laws of nutrition" apply to all of us . . . to me, and to you. Strongly entrenched food habits often overcome this point of view. We think we are well nourished, but we really are not.

Today, let's accept the challenge of planning foods for every meal, to meet the nutritional needs of our body. Let's not go beyond that point, for satisfaction of needs other than foods. With a paper and pencil, right now, plan tomorrow's meals, just day by day. Turn to the Basic Food Plan in the back of this book. Take a look at those foods needed daily by the body and plan just *one* day. You know what you have in the house, so don't plan foods that aren't familiar to you. Be certain to include protein foods, vegetables, fruits, bread, and milk (either to drink or in a recipe). Will you do it? Take one step, not later on, not maybe, not tomorrow, but right now.

This is *motivation* ... it really isn't hard, is it? When you have a day planned, give yourself a check in the box for the day at the back of the book, and every day you plan (even if it's a week ahead) take another check ... It's a rainbow day!

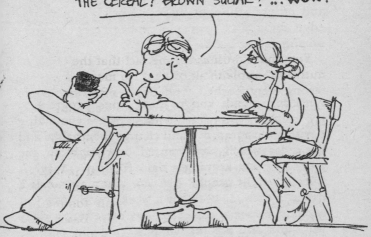

But How Much?

Let's stop again and evaluate your progress... according to your chart, what steps are you taking day by day to improve and change food habits and life-styles which have caused overweight in the past? Are you keeping a daily food inventory? A weekly weight graph? Are you planning meals a day at a time, or even for a week ahead? Are you cooking a special dish each day or setting a daily work goal and accomplishing it?

If you've taken at least three of these steps and begun to practice them daily, you're on your way; you're ready for another lesson.

Do you have a kitchen scale or a postage scale on your cupboard or near the dining table? A scale can be worth its weight in gold if you use it regularly. Protein, particularly, is an important nutrient to consider. Weigh protein foods. Obesity specialist

Dr. Jean Mayer, of Harvard University, tells us that most Americans today overeat foods with this costly ingredient (it's costly in calories as well as money).

Dr. Mayer says we would be protein-nourished with only one or two ounces of cottage cheese or one half a hamburger per day! You and I would never be able to adjust our protein-oriented habit to that, would we? Nevertheless, we can be aware of the protein-calorie count and cut down the size of our meat portions.

Let's get out that scale and weigh each portion so we really know what's happening. Let me give you some particularly good examples of various lunch proteins. You may be surprised at the low ounce recommendations. Did you know that tuna fish isn't really the lowest protein in calories, though many "diet" programs recommend it? Two ounces of tuna packed in oil contains 165 calories: the same amount of tuna with the oil drained and rinsed off is only 111. Water-packed tuna is only 72 calories per 2 ounces. What a difference that oil makes.

If you choose shrimp for lunch, 2 ounces will give you only 65 calories, one of the lowest counts you'll find. The same amount of chicken baked or broiled without skin is 77 calories, and the white meat of turkey is 100. If you're partial to veal, count 133 calories for 2 ounces; baked or broiled cod or halibut would give you 97.

Some other protein choices often recommended are cheese and cottage cheese, either as additions to the meal or for "snack foods." They, too, contain good protein nutrients, but remember to include the calories in your count. Creamed cottage cheese, for example, is 60 calories per 2 ounces; the low fat variety is only 36. Muenster cheese in a 2-ounce portion contains 200 calories, and Swiss cheese 210. These snack foods we use so often as between-meal bites are really calorie-packed monsters.

Our purpose, of course, is to encourage you to think wisely about your meats and the size of the portions you choose. You plan meals naturally, around the meat. Choose meats that will give you a lower calorie count more often than you choose the higher ones. If you're at all concerned about weight control, beef should be used only three to four times a week. Keep the amounts consumed by each member in your family lower than past habits have allowed. Your family will be well nourished, their weight will be controlled, and your grocery bill will drop. Each day you weigh the protein foods for all meals and snacks, give yourself a check in the box (see page 146) marked "Weigh" ... and have a happy ... day by day.

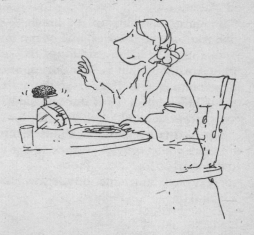

lesson eight

Body Movement

We are all resistant to change. We resist the changing seasons of the year; we deny the changing cultural standards of younger generations; sometimes we refuse to accept the fact that our weight gain is caused by changing elements in our lives.

Is it our *habit* to resist, or are these changes a complicated threat to our complacency? When we try to tackle something undefined, we face an immovable object. Isn't it possible to break down the "Impossible Dream" into little pieces and tackle them one at a time, day by day?

Although we admit food habits must change, we are often resistant to changes in body movement as well. Answer these questions realistically . . . .

Have you ever asked someone else to answer the telephone?

Have you ever said, "Will you change the TV channel while you're up?"

39

Have you ever called to one of the children, "Honey, run and get me ..."

And, let's be truthful, how often have you searched for a parking place a little closer to the store because you didn't want to walk too far?

All of these habits have an effect on our weight gains or losses. Let's look today at just how much ... or little ... we actually move our bodies. In a study at Stanford University hospital, a group of nurses were asked to wear pedometers while they walked through their daily routines. Now, nurses seem to be professionals who are constantly on the go and on their feet. To everyone's amazement these women walked less than two miles per day! Now if nurses walk so little, wouldn't it be interesting to measure the movement you and I utilize each day?

Too many are taken in by the health spa promotional pictures of glamorous men and women who are bean-pole thin. These ads imply, of course, that you can be as thin if you use the exercise machines they offer. But truthfully, you can lose the grand total of one-half pound in a year's time if you use the belt vibrator five days a week for twenty minutes at a time. A thirty to forty-five minute walk each day, however, can give you that one-half pound weight loss *each week*. Added to this benefit is the strengthening of cardiovascular functions and a feeling of well-being and relaxation.

We believe exercise is something which may easily be added to our daily Slim Life. It's a matter of programming some time into our regular routines. Decide what form of exercise, or what sport, is most acceptable to your life-style and go to it!

40

For those of us who have long been overweight, deeply ingrained personal images may have to be thoroughly shaken before we begin to expend more caloric energy. It isn't easy to move when we're programmed to sit. Some, who were overweight as children, have memories of avoiding childhood games because it was too difficult to win. Or perhaps you don't want to compete with others because you know bathing suits, leotards, and shorts weren't made for you. If this concern is holding you back from some form of body movement . . . find a conservative sports outfit and take heart. Take a simple daily walk to get you started. The whole secret is daily repetition until body movement becomes a daily habit. Your immovable object has met an irresistible force!

I personally found it necessary to keep a record of my routines. I kept a chart, similar to the one you are keeping for each chapter assignment. When I couldn't give myself a check each day, I felt badly and tried twice as hard the next day . . . but don't ever let your program go more than two days! A day after day loss is too hard to make up!

People procrastinate, "Well, I walked for five days and then it rained, so I didn't go out, and I just stopped right there." You won't melt in the rain . . . we have clothes that keep us warm and dry in any weather. Too many of us run from the house to the car, or the car to the store, and think we've been "outside." If you find you really *can't* take that daily half-hour walk, why not try running in place for ten minutes, or walking up and down the basement stairs for ten minutes, or riding a bicycle for fifteen to twenty minutes. Vary your exercise if you become bored. If you do walk, vary your route. But be consistent . . . don't just sit there . . . Do something!

Assignment: Take a half-hour walk or its equivalent each day. When you do, give yourself a check in the box on page 146. A healthier, happier, slimmer you will be your reward.

THE ROAD TO SUCCESS . . .
is marked with many tempting parking places.
—AUTHOR UNKNOWN

lesson nine

Exercise Exchanges

"I don't know why I can't lose weight. I really don't eat much. Lots of people eat more than I do, and yet I'm the one who gains!"

Does that sound familiar to you? We rationalize when we're "wishing" to lose a little weight. I say "wishing" instead of "working" because there is a difference, you know.

Let me give you an idea which might help if you're one of the slightly overweight (or more than just slightly) who has "rationalized" a time or two.

What one food do you eat every day, or twice a day, that you know contains too many calories? For example, do you allow yourself just one small chocolate chip cookie, or its caloric equivalent, each day? Isn't that a total of seven during the week? (Or maybe you ate the "whole thing" in a one-day binge.) Remember, I said "a cookie" or its equivalent. If you're not a cookie eater, think of the food in your life that is more irresistible . . . perhaps that little piece of cheese before dinner. Now . . . a small cookie contains 50 calories. That's 350 calories in a week's time, or 18,200 in a year. Since it takes 3,500 calories to lose (or add) a pound, you could gain 5 pounds a year just by eating that one cookie a day.

How can we change that habit? Give up the cookies? Yes, that's one idea, but sometimes we aren't willing to deprive ourselves. When we feel sorry for ourselves, we might substitute a habit that would cause even more trouble. So . . . if the answer for you is not to give up cookies completely, or cut the amount down effectively, you must burn off the ill effects. This you can do with little effort. A ten-minute walk or a six-minute bicycle ride will take care of that one cookie a day. While we're at it, if we increase the walk or the bike ride to twice the distance and still eat the cookie, we can lose five pounds a year, and only change the one habit!

Are you beginning to see the light, to add and subtract for yourself? What if we gave up the cookie, took a twenty-minute walk, and didn't change any other habits? Right! We'd lose ten pounds in a year's time! Dwell on that thought today, and perhaps you'll find a technique which will work for you.

There are many good books available on the subject of food and exercise exchanges. If this interests you, may I suggest Dr. Frank Konoshi's *Exercise Equivalents of Food* or Dr. Charles Kuntzelman's *Activetics*. Both books are excellent sources of ideas to increase caloric output with the idea of weight control in mind. And with each passing day, as you follow your chosen program, you'll experience new sources of energy, increased muscle tone, and a feeling of well-being. Life doesn't begin at forty, it begins when you start to care enough to care for yourself.

I find my own self-discipline is not always the strongest when I begin an exercise program. Therefore, over the years I've belonged to an exercise group at the local YMCA. When I'm with others I exercise much more vigorously than I might alone, and I enjoy it more. I have the added advantage of becoming involved in competitive sports such as racketball, volleyball, and swimming. It's fun! I've learned to love the Y and the people involved. Perhaps you might give it a try.

Assignment: Each day you can increase your caloric output by fifty calories (a half hour's walk) give yourself a big X in the box on page 146. To eat, or not to eat that cookie is no longer a question for us.

APPROXIMATE CALORIES USED UP PER HOUR BY ACTIVITIES

	120 lb. Woman	160 lb. Man
Bicycling, moderate	192	256
Bicycling, energetic	480	640
Cooking, active	96	128
Dancing, moderate	264	352
Dressing, undressing	96	128
Driving car	108	144
Eating	84	112

Exercise, moderate	240	320
Gardening, active	276	368
Golf	144	192
Housework, active	240	320
Ironing	120	160
Lying at rest	60	80
Office work, active	120	160
Painting furniture	144	192
Ping-Pong	300	400
Piano playing	132	176
Rowing	600	800
Running	444	592
Sawing wood	372	496
Sewing, knitting	84	112
Sitting at rest	84	112
Skating	252	356
Skiing	624	832
Swimming	480	640
Tennis	336	448
Typing	108	144
Walking, moderately	168	224
Writing	84	112

Remember, these figures are for a sustained hour of this activity, and so walking for a full hour may burn only 200 calories. This means that to experience weight reduction you must seriously watch your calorie consumption. You can't let yourself go and eat a lot at the next meal because you've exercised previously that day.

lesson ten

Behavior

Do you feel strong today? Are you sure enough of yourself to tackle an assignment that will assist you in controlling your weight? These studies and the research by behavioral scientists can give us some real food for thought. They tell us that overweight is not necessarily caused by some deep psychological problem. It may not be a physical thing such as inherited tendencies or underactive glands. Weight may be adversely affected simply by patterns we've learned over the years, habits of which we are not aware.

Many research programs have studied behavior habits. Dr. Richard Stuart documented the first book. Dr. Albert Stunkart pioneered in the field and Dr. Leonard Levitz and Dr. Henry Jordan, from the University of Pennsylvania, have measured results in working with overweight groups, striving to cause awareness of habits. Techniques are being developed to assist people in changing behavior. All do not work with everyone, because each of us has different stimuli that signal the desire to eat. But if one or two of these techniques helps you, it's a step forward, and all it takes is practice. What do you say? Want to give it a try today? You have only yourself to challenge, and it could be fun.

The method for today is to concentrate on trying to slow down the process of eating. It has been proven in the research projects mentioned that when we take longer to eat, we don't desire or demand as great a quantity of food.

Concentrate on only one meal a day to start. Here's the assignment: Conscientiously take a minimum of fifteen minutes' eating time for lunch each day, and no less than thirty for the evening meal.

"How in heaven's name do I do that?" Most of us gulp our meals so rapidly that our stomachs never do have time to signal back to the brain, "We have enough food, thank you." Slowing down can make us more conscious of what we are eating. We taste each food, experience the texture, and increase the pleasure. Here are some little ways to assist you in slowing the eating process.

1. Before you pick up your fork to begin eating, slowly sip a glass of water.

2. Concentrate on chewing and swallowing each mouthful before you add another bite.

3. After every fourth bite, put your fork down. Gradually work to increase this to a one-to-one ratio . . . take a bite, put down your fork, take a bite, etc.

4. Try chewing each mouthful twenty times before swallowing and adding another.

5. And, of course, take very small bites.

Sounds silly? Is it too much bother? My family would call it, "Mickey Mouse." But is it childish? To learn a new habit, we first may have to "unlearn" an old one. Or if that is too difficult, just practice, practice, practice the new one. Awareness, concentration, dedication . . . these are words we know but don't relate to food habits. Again, I ask, "Are you willing to try; do you have time to lose weight?"

Assignment: Each time you are able to concentrate on at least two of the above suggestions during the day, give yourself a check in the box. When you eat too much and eat too fast, it isn't an antacid tablet you need, it's a slow and easy life-style.

SLOW ME DOWN, LORD!
Slow me down, Lord!
Ease the pounding of my heart by the quieting of my mind.
Steady my hurried pace.
With a vision of the eternal reach of time.
Give me, amidst the confusion of my day,
The calmness of the everlasting hills.
Break the tension of my nerves
With the soothing music of the singing streams
That live in my memory.
Help me to know the magical restoring power of sleep.

49

lesson eleven

*Teach me the art of taking minute vacations of
    slowing down.
To look at a flower.
To chat with an old friend or make a new one;
To pat a stray dog; to watch a spider build a web;
To smile at a child; or to read from a good book.
Remind me each day
That the race is not always to the swift;
That there is more to life than increasing its speed.
Let me look upward into the towering oak
And know that it grew great and strong
Because it grew slowly and well.*

—ORIN L. CRAIN

lesson eleven

More Behavior

"Why me, Lord? Oh, why do I have to have a 'fat head'?" That was my daily plea. I'd reach for a doughnut or a chocolate bar and protest, "Why did You do this to me?" I'd see a slim, pretty mother with slim, pretty children and I'd cry, "Why do I have to be the fattest one at every PTA meeting?" Over the years, instead of spending time developing ways to control a "condition" for which there is no medical cure, I'd spend my time eating and moaning and groaning, "Why me?"

I believe there is no such thing as having WILL-POWER ... it's not a gift God gives some and not others. Willpower must be developed day by day and step by step. It's a slow process of learning *how* to lose weight instead of learning *what* to eat.

Remember how the baby learned to walk? He didn't just take off. There were months of creeping and crawling and tottering and holding on. Then he took that first step, holding tightly to your hand. Finally he stepped out, all on his own, into the safety of your waiting arms. Then one day, when you least expected it ... he walked, alone, across the room. And even when he fell from time to time and cried because it hurt, he got up and tried again. He didn't protest, "Why do I have to learn to walk?"

Nothing is handed to us on a silver platter. You and I must always be aware of our food habits. The sooner we accept this fact, and learn to be happy with it, the sooner our food and weight will stop becoming the most important thing in life. Life and time are far too precious for us to waste a single moment feeling sorry for ourselves. Like that baby, we'll take one step at a time ... day by day.

BUT HOW? ... let's concentrate on more behavior skills today. There are so many ideas we could choose ... but one at a time will help. Which will you work on today?

1. Don't eat anything while you are standing up.
2. Never eat while preparing or clearing up foods.
3. Choose one place which is yours and eat there only.

Assignment: Keep track of the times you use one of these techniques daily. Check the appropriate box on the chart on page 146. Remember, we're quick enough to note the failure times, but have you ever counted the times you resisted temptation and succeeded? Hooray!

Pride in our success can become a habit too, "Why NOT me?"

IF YOU THINK YOU CAN

If you think you are beaten, you are.
If you think that you dare not, you don't.
If you'd like to win, but you think you can't
It's almost certain you won't.

If you think you'll lose, you've lost,
For out in the world you'll find
SUCCESS begins with a fellow's will—
It's ALL in the state of mind.

For many a race is lost
Ere even a step is run,
And many a coward falls
Ere even his work's begun.
Think big, and your deeds will grow;
Think that you can, and you will—
It's all in the state of mind.

If you think you're outclassed, you are.
You've got to think high to rise;
You've got to be sure of yourself before
You can ever win a prize.
Life's battles don't always go
To the stronger or faster man—
But sooner or later the man who wins
Is the man who thinks he can.

—AUTHOR UNKNOWN

Slowly
Changing Habits

A delightful bit of prose struck me the other day. It's from a book by Imogene Sorley and Jo Carr, called *Bless This Mess*, and I thank them for allowing me to share some of their thoughts with you.

But, Lord, I've always bought brown sugar in square boxes with brown letters on the box.
I saw the plastic bags of sugar in the grocery store yesterday.
I could tell by looking, this was a better way. The strong, airtight bags would keep the sugar soft and usable.
BUT I'VE ALWAYS BOUGHT BROWN SUGAR IN BOXES.
And I reach for the box.
Now back home, I wonder why?
Lord, why are we ... why am I, so reluctant to change old ways?
Some old ways are valid, but some need changing.
And I cling to square boxes with unthinking tenacity;
Just because I've ALWAYS bought square boxes....

How appropriate! Isn't that the way you and I are with food habits? Don't we really cling tenaciously to old patterns... Food each time we go out! Food each time we have someone in! Food to celebrate... food for sorrow!

There is nothing you and I can do to change food habits which are centuries old. Or is there? If I'm willing to try... if I have the courage... if I want to achieve my goal of controlled weight badly enough, *I will take that step.*

But what can I do? There are several alternatives. If we can't change other people and food occasions, could we change the amounts served? Could we substitute food with low caloric count so that the results are not so devastating to our health and our figures? Are there small habits we could change? It isn't easy, but it's worth the effort.

The story ends:

> The container that brown sugar comes in is no great thing;
> But neither are other, weightier matters that require rethinking...
> And perhaps revising. If I am going to live significantly,
> I must make my big decision, purposefully... intentionally...comprehensively...

Now what steps can we take today? Is there an old habit we can change? Here are six ideas for you to practice. Each will help to keep food out of sight and reduce the eating occasions. Day by day, as you accomplish at least two of these techniques, give yourself a check in the appropriate box.

1. Choose a specific place in one room of your home to do all your eating. Use it for all meals and snacks. It may be a different place for each meal if you like. If you eat at work, avoid eating at your desk. At a restaurant, sit at your favorite table. I want your eating place to be special. Take your time, enjoy yourself, make eating a luxury and a pleasure.

2. If you eat at a regular table, change your habitual eating place. It may be less effective and it need not be forever, but break up some long-standing patterns.

3. Concentrate on eating only. Don't read or watch TV. Think about the taste of the food, how good it is . . . Enjoy the people around you.

4. Remove the serving dishes with extra foods from the table. Better yet, serve the plates in the kitchen.

5. Have lots of low-calorie foods available and in sight. When you're in the kitchen, keep dishes of cut up low-calorie vegetables and fruit right on the counter. Chew sugarless gum. Drink water or low-cal beverages.

6. Cover tempting high-calorie leftovers with foil or plastic covers. Low-cal foods should be visible in the front of the cupboard or refrigerator. Rearrange your shelves so the high-cal snacks are harder to reach. Better yet, don't keep these foods in the house.

Remember, you can't do it all at once . . . take one step at a time. Develop habits which will last and make you aware of what you are doing . . . Check your chart each day you accomplish two ideas. Think thin . . . it will work.

lesson thirteen

Changing Thoughts

This week, I studied the ideas of a psychiatrist, dealing with the emotional state of us "fat heads." I'd like to share his thoughts and some of my own. This doctor thinks the most important asset in successful weight loss is a stable control of the "anxiety" periods in our lives. He tells us that attempting to lose weight when conditions in life are full of stress is next to impossible.

But I've found the habitual dieter always enjoys some sort of emotional stress. If we don't have some handy, we're very good at manufacturing situations that "just might" happen, so we are prepared at all times by eating "good food," just in case!

Anxiety can be caused by dwelling on things which *have* happened or *might* happen. Let's see what you and I can do to keep our emotional state more stable. Let's concentrate on a happy life, happy relationships, and happy *slim* food habits.

First, consider the things which have already happened. How often do we blame ourselves or other people, or other *things*, for stressful situations? We repeat over and over again: "*If only. If only* ... I had known. If only ... they wouldn't. If only ... it hadn't happened ... *If only.*" Once an event has occurred, we cannot benefit one bit from all the "if only's" in the world. How much better it would be if we looked ahead to positive steps we might take, and substituted the words ... "Next time." See how much it helps. Instead of, "*If only* I hadn't eaten that cookie," try saying, "*Next time* I feel like eating a cookie, I'll sit right down and cut an apple into little pieces and eat them, very slowly, one at a time." What an uplift you get from planning ahead instead of looking behind!

Now, let's pounce on those events which just "might happen." Do you realize that 75 percent or more of all the thoughts we have are negative? Wow! What a percentage! Stop and think about it now. Those destructive thoughts about yourself and the possibility of failure; the paralyzing thoughts of family catastrophes caused by illness, or accidents ... are efforts in futility.

Less than 5 percent of these negative thoughts we cuddle protectively ever really happen! Do you question the word "cuddle" in reference to negative thoughts? Think again ... those negative feelings give us the opportunity to pacify ourselves in retaliation for all of the "bad" things in our life. How often that pacifier is food! STOP! When you are thinking down, replace that thought with one that's wholesome, healthy, and happy. Pick up your Bible. By reading God's Word you will always find some reason to give thanks. How much brighter the day will seem, and how unimportant the "food crutch" will become.

Task for today . . . try to eliminate, or at least recognize negative attitudes. Think logically about it . . . turn it around. Don't let it become a food excuse. Day by day, as you succeed, give yourself a check in the appropriate box on page 146.

Concentrate instead on beautiful thoughts, and cuddle those close to your heart. When I close my day, I ask the Lord to make me happy with what I have done with it. For these twenty-four hours come but once, and I can never have them to relive again. "I ask Thee, Lord, to give me a task to do today, and the courage to do it. Amen."

GOD'S KIND CARE

God hath not promised
Skies always blue,
Flower-strewn pathways,
All our lives thro';
God hath not promised
Sun without rain,
Joy without sorrow,
Peace without pain.

God hath not promised
We shall not know
Toil and temptation,
Trouble and woe;
He hath not told us
We shall not bear
Many a burden,
Many a care.

59

God hath not promised
  Smooth roads and wide,
Swift, easy travel,
  Needing no guide;
Never a mountain,
  Rocky and steep,
Never a river
  Turbid and deep:

But God hath promised
  Strength for the day,
Rest for the labor,
  Light for the way,
Grace for the trials,
  Help from above,
Unfailing sympathy,
  Undying love.

—ANNIE JOHNSON FLINT

lesson fourteen

Relax,
It's Good for You!

Is anything more soothing than the squeak of a
rocking chair as you rhythmically relax at the end
of a long and tiring day? John F. Kennedy always
kept one in the Oval Office at the White House.
He would "sit a spell" and relax physically while
his active mind absorbed world problems.

Relaxation is an art that needs time and concentration to develop. We spend hours working for
our family and others, and even more time thinking about all we have to do. Relaxation and positive
thought will make it even easier to accomplish
difficult tasks.

I played a cassette tape the other day. The title,
"How to Lose Weight," suggested great words of
wisdom from an expert with a magic key. (Don't we
all look for the Magic Key?) Instead, I heard a re-
laxing experience. Too many unhappy eating

experiences, paradoxically, actually result from worry about overeating and avoiding certain foods. As a result, we "concentrate" ourselves right into the food. If we relaxed a bit, then approached the problem, we might feel differently about it.

When you feel so terribly tired or hassled and busy, do you say, "I'll have something to eat and then I can finish what I have to do"? We're all guilty! Next time, stop before you take that first bite, lie down for ten minutes, and then decide whether or not you still want food. Surprisingly, you may not need it. Take time to rest; all you'll gain is energy.

Try this assignment at least once each day this week. Come on now, you can do it. Sit or lie down and take a deep breath. Close your eyes and take an even deeper breath. Let your hands relax . . . and then your feet. Now relax your body from the toes up, one at a time. Focus all of your attention on one limb, wiggle it just a bit, feel the tension leave, and relax . . .

Begin with the toes . . . relax the big one, the next one, and right on down. Now concentrate on the calves . . . relax . . . relax. The thighs, the hips. Relax . . . relax . . .

Ready to move on? Relax the stomach, the abdomen, the waist. Think your way up your back, one vertebra at a time. Relax across the chest, and relax the shoulders . . . Now down the right arm, to the hands, each finger, one at a time. Try the left arm the same way. Reach the neck and the face, the lips, the nose, the eyes, the top of your head. Relax . . . lie there . . . sit there . . . Just relax. Breathe deeply. Again. Now, very slowly open your eyes, and smile.

62

How do you feel? Read it again and again until you learn the routine. Promise yourself you'll slow down in this manner at least once a day this week. How good you'll feel when you relax. Each day you repeat the routine at least once, give yourself a check. Take it easy . . . Relax.

Just close your eyes and open your heart,
And feel your cares and worries depart;
Just yield yourself to the Father above
And let Him hold you secure in His love.
—HELEN STEINER RICE

lesson fifteen

Appearance

"From this day on . . . I will not feel sorry for myself, I will not pamper myself with food; and day by day, I will try to make myself more attractive." That's our thought for today.

We must realize that our attitude toward proper foods and weight control are keynotes to our day-to-day life. Just what is your attitude toward yourself today? Do you feel attractive? What can you and I do to increase our self-confidence? Let's look at some answers together.

Everything we do has a bearing on our personal feelings of self-worth. Did you know that you smile more often when you're slim? When you're losing weight you have a reason to smile! Walk down the street and catch a glimpse of your reflection in a store window; you'll smile. The slimmer you become, the quicker the smile will come. People enjoy being near a person who laughs readily, but you and I know well that a laugh on the outside covers a cry from inside a fat body. As we slim down, we build self-assurance within.

The way we walk and stand and carry ourselves reflects an inner source, or lack, of self-reliance. Remember the song's observation, "There's a kind of walk you walk when you're feeling happy... There's a kind of walk you walk when you're feeling sad." Practice projecting the image you want others to see. Look into the mirror and smile... come on, now, don't be shy! Stand tall and straight ... walk happy. You'll find you've put your best foot forward, physically and literally.

Now look at your hands. A dead giveaway to a fat mind are the arms and hands crossed over the fat tummy. We think we've covered up some of the hated fat, but really we've only called attention to it. What can we do with those flapping fingers on the ends of our arms? Hold them behind... in front... at the side... use them to gesture? Why not perform for yourself as gracefully as possible in front of the full-length mirror. Be a bit of a ham ... gestures can be beautifully expressive... see how you look, and practice using your hands effectively.

Clothing and outward appearance help build our sense of self-pride. As we grow slimmer and more attractive, we find it's a pleasure to shop and treat ourselves to something new. In one Slim Living class, a woman told me she bought herself a new dress after I had told her the week before to treat herself as important. That's a splendid idea. If you're not ready to buy, try on something new and set a goal for the future. And always remodel your clothing as it becomes too loose-fitting. It may be funny when someone calls you "baggy pants," but you'll look slimmer faster with sagging seams taken in a bit. Skirts tend to droop in back as the hips reduce, and trousers develop pleats whether that's the cut or not.

Don't forget that men's clothing today comes in flattering new styles and bright, attractive colors, but rarely in extra-extra large sizes. And what a metamorphosis men's hairstyles have undergone. Keep up with the changes for your own pride's sake. Do you have the confidence to change? Perhaps a styled cut or a groomed mustache or beard might be just right for you, men.

We women need to take critical looks at new hairstyles and makeup as well. I visit my makeup consultant periodically just to ask what's new in colors and styles. I don't try to adhere to all trends, but I do like to know what's current, and a new shade of lipstick works wonders for my self-image and morale. How about you? Do you have the nerve to try some of the latest hairstyles and make-up tricks; have you worn the same look for too many years?

Ask yourself these questions and then decide if your attitude toward yourself needs changing.

1. When is the last time you bought something new to wear?
2. Was it a smaller or larger size than you bought the time before?
3. How do you react if the sales clerk tells you that you look so "small," and you feel you're not? Do you tense up?

4. Are you confident enough of yourself to walk up to people and talk at a social event, or do you wait for them to come to you?
5. Have your eating habits changed so that you're more aware, not only of calories, but also of nutrients?
6. What are you planning to do this week to make yourself more attractive day by day?

Assignment for this lesson: Evaluate your personal appearance and your attitude toward yourself. If you make some small change, give yourself a check in the appropriate box.

Remember: Smile, and the world smiles with you; cry, and you use a lot of tissues.

lesson sixteen

Cook
Something Special

The sun is shining and I feel light and lovely inside today. That's where it starts, you know. The mood I'm in, the things I have to do . . . definitely affect the foods I eat. If it's gloomy, and there is nothing I'll enjoy doing on the day's schedule . . . wow, look out sweets! If I feel insecure " 'cause nobody loves me," my cravings lean toward meats and breads. Funny, but that's the way it goes.

But . . . today, the sun is shining, inside and out. It's the kind of day that helps me face the kitchen and cooking with a creative mind and a light caloric touch. Let me share what I plan to cook and perhaps you'd like to cook light and lovely, too.

Frozen Snack Treat

1/2 cup crushed pineapple packed in its own
    juice
1/3 cup powdered milk
1 tsp. flavoring
A few drops sweetener if desired
Stir together, place in small shallow dish.
Freeze. Cut and eat.

I enjoy using chocolate extract and brown food
color, or coconut extract, or orange, or banana, or
tropical fruit. Try your favorite.

Pineapple Cardamom Cookies

1/4 cup crushed pineapple
2/3 cup milk powder
1 tsp. coconut extract
1/2 tsp. cardamom or coriander
    (use nutmeg instead if you prefer)
Sweetener to taste

Be certain pineapple is well drained. You might
care to add 1 T. raisins and 6 chopped walnuts.
Drop by the teaspoonful onto Pam-sprayed pan.
Bake at 350 degrees for about 15 minutes. They're
great!

Mother's Chicken Broth with Vegetables

Simmer one chicken till done. Remove meat
(save for another meal), place broth in refrigerator
till fat is congealed at top and can be removed. Add
diced celery, green beans, peas and carrots, onion,
pimiento or red pepper, cauliflower (whatever
vegetable your refrigerator will yield) and simmer
slowly till vegetables are soft. Enjoy this soup any-
time for a wonderful homemade taste.

By now, you understand today's assignment. Cook something special for yourself. It doesn't have to take a long time. It needn't be a gourmet dish. A simple treat like a low-cal malt in the blender can make you feel like a queen or king. Just knowing that it's a treat and it's for you alone will give you a warm, shiny glow. *Do it now* . . . and then put a check in the box for today on your score sheet. Look at those checks! Each one shows that you *do care* about your weight, and more than that, you're doing something about it. How many checks for today?

lesson seventeen

Fluids Help, Too

What importance do fluids play in our everyday weight life? Many people, men and women, have a tremendous problem with body retention of fluids. They have a fear of drinking water in large quantities, but the same people may have no concern when it comes to other beverages—coffee, tea, pop, or alcohol. Let's talk about the problem.

There are several ways to test your tendencies toward fluid retention. If your rings seem tight and your fingers or feet swell, it could be a sign. If your weight fluctuates four to eight pounds within a day, it might be a symptom. You may look puffy around the eyes. Place your thumb on the inner ankle bone, move it two inches up the leg and, with one thumb on top of the other, press firmly. You can determine the excess fluid in your body by the deepness of the indentation, the severe discoloration, or the length of time before the hollow is filled again.

Fluid retention will not keep you from losing weight, but it does slow down the process, and that's discouraging when your food intake is under control. In this case, I encourage you to weigh yourself just once a week, at the same time each week. Take measurements of your body every four weeks to compare changes and losses.

Instead of avoiding water when your body is swollen with fluids, quite the opposite is necessary. To help your body flush out the waste products you have accumulated while burning fat, it is more necessary than ever that you drink water. We suggest four to eight glasses a day to our classes. Other fluids help, but they ofte contain additional unwanted properties. Suga -free beverages, for instance, contain a great deal of sodium to improve the flavor. If you retain fluids, what you don't need is more sodium. Instant coffee also contains sodium, and nutritionists suggest the possibility that coffee may lower the blood sugar and accelerate feelings of hunger.

Many foods will cause you to retain fluids, if you have that tendency. Hot dogs, sauerkraut, dill pickles, even celery, contain a great deal of salt which accelerates the problem of fluid retention. Other foods act as natural diuretics. Foods containing iodine are helpful, since that mineral is one regulator for fluid in the cells and tissues. These include anything from the sea . . . fish of all varieties, spinach, iodized salt, etc. But drinking enough water daily is the easiest and best suggestion.

Assignment for the day: Can you strive to drink a minimum of four glasses of water daily? Each time you do, mark it on your chart (see page 146). Remember, eat (low calorie foods), drink (lots of water), and be merry!

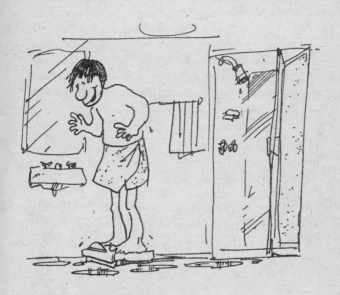

lesson eighteen

"Cold Turkey"

Have you ever heard of "Cold Turkey"? I don't mean the kind you have after a holiday ... what we're talking about is more comparable to withdrawal from drugs or alcohol.

Already you're saying, "This crazy woman wants me to fast, with no food at all: I'm not going to do it!" No, I would never suggest that you go without any food at all. That's what makes this "controlling-my-weight" racket so difficult. We must have food to survive. We simply cannot go into complete withdrawal. However, there is something to be said for withdrawal from a certain food form.

Suppose you and I make the decision that, for the next three weeks, we withdraw completely from foods which contain sugar. I'm not including natural sugars already in fruits or vegetables, or even the bit added to breads which makes the yeast activate. You know the foods I mean. The very name could trigger a salient food response in you.

What happens to the body when we withdraw from sugar for this length of time? Well, the hypothalamus gland becomes adjusted to a lower level of sugar intake. It begins demanding less for body functions and storing of fats; thus the physical demand for these foods becomes much less as time goes on. Day by day it becomes easier to do physically. Your body may even reject sweets after a period without them, and you may find yourself a little physically ill when you next consume any amount of sugar. That doesn't mean you won't want it; we're talking about physiological demands, not psychological desires. Your "fat-eyeball" mind may still light up at the sight of a scrumptious, gooey dessert, but your body's desires will be less, and that's a help.

Just think of the people you'll be pleasing! Your dentist will be happy if you're able to cut your sugar intake. Your physician will be pleased to see your weight dropping (that happens when you cut sweet consumption). Your tailor or clothier will be pleased (you'll need a complete new wardrobe of smaller clothes). Your friends will be envious; that's not all bad, for it may just encourage them to do the same. Your spouse, or your family, may have some changes in attitude toward you; and, as your weight goes down, I'm betting your attitude toward yourself will change as well.

What about it? . . . Is it worth three weeks of "Cold Turkey" to begin a sensible *weigh* of life? Each day you conscientiously feel you have gone without any added sugar, mark yourself an "X" on the chart. A "sweet-less" you will become a "sweeter" you.

lesson nineteen

Vegetables...
Ugh...

Ah, those happy days of summer, when vegetables and fruits abound and living is slim and easy! What a shame that our grandparents enjoyed fresh vegetables only in the good old summertime. Perhaps if the fresh ones had been as available as they are now, you and I might have inherited a greater taste for these healthful, calorie-cutting, tasty morsels. As it is, the most ignored foods in our American diets are vegetables. Nutritionists speak of the vegetable as the "golden food" of good health and weight control.

Children will imitate the vegetable habits of their families. Consider your likes and dislikes. Are they similar to those of your parents? And how about your own family? At the table does Daddy say, "No vegetables," and do the children echo, "Me, either!"? Is Mother so unaccustomed to being creative with vegetables that she opens a can of peas or corn and says, "Eat, it's good for you!"

These luscious nuggets, so loaded with the vitamins and minerals we need for good health and growth, should be routinely included in our daily menus. Our generation benefits from the latest shipping, packing, and freezing methods. The variety of vegetables is endless, and frozen food companies creatively entice us with exotic combinations that have taste and eye appeal. But do resist those combinations which have high caloric sauces if you're working toward good weight control.

Many brands in your local supermarket are packed without heavy sauces. If you can't find them, you can always mix tempting varieties yourself, using commercial packages for starters. Browse a bit and see if you can create a combination or two for this week. Let the whole family help with planning and suggestions. Offer a special prize for the combination the family votes their favorite for the week.

TRY:

1. peas, green beans, celery, and red pepper
2. summer squash or zucchini, tomatoes, onions
3. carrots, broccoli, onions
4. water chestnuts, bean sprouts, carrots, mushrooms
5. summer squash with apple or pineapple
6. cabbage, green pepper, onion
7. celery braised in tomato juice
8. cauliflower, carrots, green pepper, pimiento
9. French style green beans, onion, mushrooms

10. broccoli, green onions, mushrooms, one potato
11. carrots and onions
12. sauerkraut, celery, green pepper, pimiento
13. carrots and pineapple
14. acorn squash stuffed with applesauce
15. asparagus and mushrooms
16. beets, pineapple, oranges

Season each combination wisely and turn the family on to a whole new taste treat.

Assignment for the day: Try a new vegetable idea. Each day you do . . . give yourself a check on your daily chart. You, too, can turn the lowly vegetable into a gourmet dish fit for a royal family— your own. Be colorfully creative . . . begin with vegetables.

lesson twenty

The Nutrition Game

Nutrition ... what does that word do for you? It sounds boring and scholarly if you're having a dull day. But our days are not dull, so we'll spell the word, "newtrition." "New" ideas are always fun, and we can make a game out of a dull word for all in the family to try. New slogans help us learn more about new food categories. Learn the slogans, then give the key word and see what new letter combinations each one can suggest.

"Carbohydrates are not cool" ... they burn and give us energy. The foods such as bread and cereal and sugar and sweets are warm and secure. They provide heat and energy for our bodies. We need carbohydrates, but we must limit them if we want to control our weight.

"Protein protects" ... that's right, it protects us against diseases; it builds and repairs our body tissues, bone, skin, hair, and blood. It's found in strong foods such as meat, fish, poultry, eggs, and milk. We need protein every day, but not to excess if we are to remain slim.

"Fat is flabby" . . . Fat bodies are flabby, and fat foods are flabby. Butter, oil, shortenings, bacon, chocolate, nuts, and meats are full of flabby fat. Fat staves off hunger, and some fat helps the skin, but use it sparingly.

Now do you understand our game? Try it again. "Carbohydrates _____" . . . "Fat is_____" . . . "Protein _____." . . . Good! Now try some minerals and vitamins.

"Calcium can be chilled" . . . Milk and cheese and sardines and shellfish, and even green leafy vegetables such as spinach, contain calcium and need refrigeration. Calcium builds strong bones and fine, white teeth.

"Iron has strength" . . . It builds red blood and strong muscles. We find it in strong foods, like meat, liver, egg yolk, dried fruits, and whole grains.

"Phosphorus preserves" . . . good healthy bones and teeth. Meat, fish, poultry, dried peas and beans, milk and milk products, egg yolk, and whole grain bread and cereals all provide perfect phosphorus.

"Iodine is important" . . . It's just a minute mineral; there are only about twelve grains in our bodies, but iodine is necessary for the *function* of the thyroid gland. Seafoods, iodized salt, and some vegetables give us "important iodine."

"Thiamine's tasty" . . . and it promotes good appetite and digestion. What is the source of thiamine? Tasty, whole grains.

"Riboflavin's right on" ... to keep our vision clear, oxygen in our cells, and our skin smooth. Good sources are milk, liver, cheese, and green, leafy vegetables.

"Niacin is necessary" ... for appetite and good nerves. We'll find it in those necessary foods: vegetables, whole grains.

"Vitamin C is in Citrus" ... Don't think of oranges and grapefruit as the only sources of vitamin C. Remember that strawberries, tomatoes, broccoli, cabbage, melons, and even potatoes contain vitamin C. Why do we need it? It helps us resist infection and binds the cells and walls of blood vessels together. Let's not fall apart!

"Vitamin A keeps us alert" ... It's good for eyes and skin, and helps us resist infection. Once again, liver, fish, dark green, leafy vegetables, yellow fruits, and vegetables are sources.

"Vitamin D is demanded" ... by our body for bones and teeth. It's abundantly supplied by milk, liver, fish, and egg yolk.

Begin with just these fun slogans. Add ideas of your own to the game. Now look again; did you note the repetition of important foods which we must include in our "day by day" menus? Today's assignment: Look ahead for one week and see if your family food plan includes some of the foods in each of your game categories. If you're following the Basic Slim Living Plan, the food groups will be included—but remember that variety is the spice of a slim life. Even a good plan can be boring if you neglect creativity. Give yourself a check whenever you play the "newtrition game." It's the ABC's of happiness and good health.

Thank you, Lord, for this body . . .
For the wondrous things it can perform.
Teach me to treat it respectfully
To your glory till you shall transform.

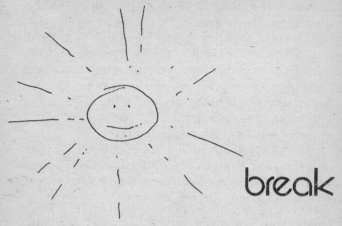

break

STOP! It's time to evaluate. Now that you've read the previous pages carefully, you know what your problems are and you know there are solutions just waiting for you to try. Some ideas will be more helpful than others. Use them . . . faithfully . . . and don't give up. Remember the little engine that said, "I think I can . . . I think I can"? And he could; *so can you.*

It's time now to look ahead and prepare ourselves to answer those tricky questions we may face tomorrow . . . or the day after that.

lesson twenty-one

What Will Today Bring?

Welcome to the great "lending library in the sky." Maybe you already belong to the club. A friend says, "Have you read . . . ," and you exchange ideas from the latest diet book or a recent Erma Bombeck satire. It's fun and it's a good way to be conversationally current.

I enjoy reading every book or article which talks about weight control. At first I thought the more I read, the more I'd lose. Then I discovered that eating ice cream while I read didn't help one bit. Nevertheless, I find that reading about new ideas helps me to be more aware. Even the kookiest of fad books has one or two sections which make sense or have some philosophic value . . . and, I'm prepared when someone says, "Have you read . . . ?"

Have you read the books by Jo Carr and Imogene Sorley? My favorite is *Prayers for People Who*

Are Too Busy Not to Pray. Over and over again their happy thoughts guide me through the difficult places . . . out of corners I had labeled "no way out." I relate my "fat food" self to every one of their situations. How it helps to have a prayerful friend.

Behavioral scientists tell us that overweight people are expertly adept at premeditating food disasters. Oh, that hurts! And just when I was thinking, "I suppose I'll blow the diet this weekend. I've got to go to the party, it's my husband's birthday." We really do plan disasters before they ever happen. It's known as a subterfuge . . . an elaborate plan of blaming someone or something else for our shortcomings. Super sleuths and arch-criminals should have the minds of you and me, the "fat heads," when it comes to maneuvering a face to face confrontation with our food favorites!

Oh, the excuses I can think of right now for this weekend! "I've worked hard this week and I deserve a treat." "He'll be upset if I don't eat some birthday cake." "I can't say 'no' to food at a party; what will *they* think?" "I'll be extra good next week so I can have *fun* . . . this week." Such clever excuses; how do you fantasize?

The point is, the busier we are, the more we need to plan in advance, to pray, to be ready. Perhaps you and I can be executive managers in our lives, day by day. Add this to your list.

Learn to plan one food event a day. Ask yourself early in the morning, "What will be my most difficult food test today?" Will it be a time of day, a busy period when foods must be grabbed and consumed? Will it be an event . . . a party, a meal out?

Will it be simply not taking time to plan a meal? We talked before about meal planning one day at a time. Go a step further and look into those events and situations we could preplan.

For instance, you've been invited to an open house tonight from five to six o'clock. You know there will be snack foods and beverages available, but no proper meal. What are the alternatives?

1. Abstain . . . simply don't eat anything.
2. Take or ask for a low-calorie beverage and keep your hands full.
3. Stand away from food tables and concentrate on conversations with people rather than on food.
4. Eat a low-cal salad before going.
5. Plan exactly what you will eat when you leave the party, and have it ready so you don't become excessively hungry.
6. If you decide you are going to eat, plan ahead exactly what and how much.

Try walking yourself through the situation mentally, step by step, and try to anticipate what might happen.

Plan just one event a day, or one meal . . . and place a check of success in the appropriate box on your chart. Are you ready? As Mother used to say, "A stitch in time saves a lot of embarrassment."

lesson twenty-two

Preplanning

Have you read *Alice in Wonderland*? Did you see the Walt Disney production? Remember the song the White Rabbit sings, "I'm late, I'm late for a very important date!"? That song sums up my life some days. Some days! What am I talking about? Every day! How about you?

Do you realize that such hustle and bustle is a perfect excuse for you and me to ignore our food routine, not taking time to plan, or cook, or eat wisely?

What's your day-by-day schedule? Up at seven or before, hurry through breakfast, and get everyone on his way? If you're a woman, you're concerned about your family . . . you know they need a good breakfast to maintain good health. If you're a man, you're rushing to punch a time clock, or keep an appointment. You shower and dress—

hurry, hurry, get everything in order . . . dash out of the house to work, to the market, or to chauffeur the family somewhere. Day by day, you've an unending list of very important dates . . . and you're late.

With such a hectic schedule, what do you have for breakfast? Stand-up toast and coffee? That won't start your day with sufficient energy and nutrients to keep you going efficiently. As a result, you find yourself grabbing a sweet roll or doughnut at coffee-break time, just because you didn't eat enough breakfast to prevent that ten A.M. slump. Sooner or later your weight begins to climb. Admit it, then do something about it.

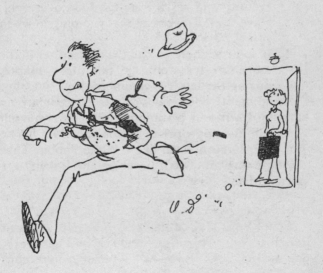

Let's tackle two ideas, for it's never too late to change bad habits. Remember, if we choose one or two suggestions each day and concentrate on them, we're progressing toward our goal. Let's break the rush-rush habit. Let's save time for an adequate breakfast and time to plan for the day. Eating a better breakfast may require a complete reorganization of your day-by-day routine. Good . . . a new schedule means a new you.

One or more of these suggestions might help:

1. Get up fifteen minutes earlier. Sit down and enjoy a breakfast centered around the ideas in the basic food plan.
2. Pack lunches for yourself or the family in the evening and refrigerate the food overnight.
3. Have the coffeepot all ready to plug in when you get up.
4. If you routinely unload the dishwasher in the morning, try doing it the night before, during the last TV commercial.

Assignment: Each day you can concentrate on slowing down and planning ahead, give yourself a check in the appropriate box on page 146. It's no fun to rush, rush, rush like a White Rabbit. Take the time to plan. You'll never be late for any important date.

lesson twenty-three

Rewards and Incentives

"New . . . exciting . . . revolutionary!" Many market products advertise a change of ingredients frequently just so they can promote those very words! We Americans search constantly for something new and exciting. We're quickly bored with anything old, used, and trite. Even in our food habits, we look for exotic new ideas that are easy and quick to prepare.

Have you watched the growth of the fast-food shops? From hamburger chains, to fried chicken and fried fish, to pizza and tacos . . . we've loved every new fad. How can we calorie-conscious adults resist?

We know we can't try everything, then grab a pill or a shot or a candy to protect us from the consequences. Yet we, too, yearn for the excitement of new ideas. To keep our motives strong, we need to work for specifics. That's what will add excitement and the feeling of playing a new game. The basic, underlying thought, however, is always good, sensible eating ideas.

While you try the motivational ideas in this chapter, be constantly aware that each day you must have the basic four ... bread and cereals, fruits and vegetables, milk, and meats.

Let's set up a system of awards to use in the weeks ahead. I don't mean plans such as: "When I lose five pounds, I'll have a banana split." Make it something unrelated to food ... something fun and rewarding that makes you feel proud. Many of us are motivated by money. In one weight-loss clinic the patient contracts with his caseworker at the beginning of treatment. The patient agrees to lose a certain amount within a certain time period. One hundred dollars is deposited by the patient. At the end of the period, if the patient has lost the specified amount, fifty dollars is returned to him. The balance is not returned until a year from that date. If the weight is still off, the patient receives the rest of his money ... if he defaults at either point, the money is kept by the therapist. Now that takes real courage.

I won't ask you to send me one hundred dollars in small bills for motivation. Instead, I'll give you a system which works for me when I need a motivational boot. For many of my rewards, I ask the cooperation of my family. Since it is much easier to control weight with the help of another, I discuss my plans with them.

Some of my rewards are money-related; many more are time-related. Several are things I personally enjoy doing, but resist when I know there is other work to be done. As you read my motivation list, think of things which interest you. Granted, most suggestions could be done without earning points, but it's more fun and exciting when I count my self-worth as I earn my rewards.

Two steps are necessary. First, set a schedule of points you may earn. Put them in a point bank to spend later as you desire. Keep as many points as you wish and spend them whenever you wish. It's important to have small and large rewards as incentives to keep you going.

Next, you must set up a series of awards. Add new ideas as you go along. I keep a daily total of what I have earned and a running account of my bank balance as I spend points.

SCHEDULE...TO EARN AND BANK POINTS
1. A very good nutritious meal .... 3 points
2. An excellent food day ....12 points
3. 7 good food days in a row ..500 bonus points
4. To cook a special food ....25 points
5. To bike 5 minutes ....15 points
6. To walk 20 minutes ....25 points
7. To exercise 10 minutes ....20 points
8. No snacks between 3:30 & 6:00 P.M. 50 points
9. To resist a fat food ....10 points
10. To slow down ....10 points
11. To plan a day ahead ....25 points
12. To keep a food inventory for the day 20 points
13. To prepare special vegetables ......25 points
14. To drink 4 glasses of water daily ...25 points

SCHEDULE ... TO SPEND POINTS

1. To buy a plant ....50 points
2. Take a bubble bath ....25 points
3. To read for one hour uninterrupted 50 points
4. To sew for an hour uninterrupted ..50 points
5. To buy something for $2 ....100 points
6. To buy something for $5 ....250 points
7. To make or buy a new article of clothing
   ....500 points
8. To have lunch with a friend ......50 points
9. To enjoy a day at my YMCA health club,
   a massage included ....150 points
10. To place flowers in my home .....200 points
11. To make myself a low-cal shake ...100 points
12. A very special treat, a weekend trip
    ....3000 points

Now, what can you think of that interests you? Does the idea appeal to your sporting nature? I challenge you to try it for two weeks and see if it doesn't help. Give yourself a check in the box every day you record points. Remember, there's no punishment for failing; we punish ourselves enough when things go wrong. There is only reward for developing good habits. Why not give it a try today? It will help you along your road to good health and a Slim Life ... and that in itself will be new, exciting, and perhaps revolutionary.

lesson twenty·four

The Good Deeds Jar

Someone said to me at a party, "I can't eat that cake, I've given up sweets for Lent. I'm going to lose a few pounds before Easter, too."

I was momentarily startled to discover that her self-denial for the Lenten season had an "ulterior" motive. It was a two-for-one bargain. Many things we do for others give us a "payoff" as well. That's good! We need a reward for a goal accomplished, and that reward might well be just "feeling good."

Most Christian circles today emphasize services to others instead of self-denial. And . . . if we utilize this service for a twofold purpose, perhaps it will serve us even better. Why not combine our altruistic desires with our self-seeking desire for gratification? Let's treat ourselves with service instead of with food.

The next time you wander into the kitchen,

searching the cupboards or refrigerator for something new and satisfying, stop before you reach for a "goody." Instead of food, why not take a "goody" from the "Good Deeds Jar." It's a different kind of satisfaction.

"What's the Good Deeds Jar?" you ask. That's the one we're going to make right now. You'll need a small jar, a pen, and a dozen little slips of paper to write on. Now, think of people you know who need a service you could provide, something that would take only a small portion of your time.

There's a dear older lady on our street who is paralyzed from a stroke. I haven't visited her because I didn't know what to say. I'll put that down. I know she's lonesome . . . And my mother's basement needs cleaning. That's really a good deed . . . A new family moved into the next block. I could take a bouquet from the garden. I only met them once . . . A lady from our church was just widowed; a half-hour visit would be a help . . . Old Bill, all alone, just loves to talk about his farm. My ears could listen for half an hour or so . . . I could baby-sit for an afternoon with my neighbor's four-year-old; then she could get out, and it might be fun for me, too . . . I could have lunch with that retired schoolteacher who's all alone. She loves to get out and meet friends and former students . . . I have an ivy plant started from a slip; perhaps the new mother in the next block might enjoy that. You men can think of people alone who need help with little chores that seem so big when you don't know how to do them.

There's our beginning, but go on. Bake a lemon pie for the minister's family; I know it's his favorite. Why do I always think of sweet treats? Maybe a casserole or a lovely salad creation would be better. Who ever invites a family with five children over for dinner? I *could* do it if I tried. That lady I used to work with is retired now. I wonder what she's doing? A phone call might help, and I'd enjoy talking with her. The delightful gentleman down the street who has the woodworking shop in his basement—he loves to have people look at the clever things he makes. Maybe he has a new birdhouse for the chickadees at our bird feeder. Perhaps they'd nest next spring in a new house.

As the good ideas keep coming, write them down and put them into your "Good Deeds Jar." Take one out when you're tempted to eat; indulge in time rather than calories.

To add another dimension ... try a second jar. I call it the "Put-it-off Jar," for all the tasks that I keep overlooking, those little things I never have time for. My "junk drawer" always needs cleaning ... the buttons on Jack's favorite shirt are loose ... the refrigerator needs attention ... I should clip the dog's toenails or replant the Boston fern or clean "that" closet ... repair the electrical extension cord ... clean the sewing machine. What an endless list there seems to be!

Now the idea is ... when I feel restless and know that food and I are heading toward a collision course, I go to my jars, which I keep *outside* the kitchen, and I take out a slip. Either I get a "payoff" by choosing something from the "Good Deeds Jar," or I get a warm feeling of accomplishment from one of the tasks in the "Put-it-off Jar." Then I dip my hand into the proper jar and follow through on whatever I pull out. It's exciting for me! It's a change for you ... it's a game of life, and you can play day by day.

Assignment for today: Put together your own special jars. When you do, give yourself a point on your chart. Any day you utilize this technique, put another check on the sheet! In this game, you'll always be a winner.

> *So long as we love, we serve; so long as we are loved by others, I should say that we are almost indispensable; and no man is useless while he has a friend.*

> —ROBERT LOUIS STEVENSON

lesson twenty-five

Family Involvement

No one can lose weight alone! It takes the support of those around you and control of your environment to assure weight loss and maintaining. Our lives are influenced most by our families and friends. They provide our source of reinforcement and reward. They compliment us, notice the changes, and "feedback" verbal and nonverbal opinions. The more they know about our goals the better. Some of the things we've tried may seem silly, but if those near us understand each attempt, they will help us to be more effective.

Our families and friends need to know the importance we place on weight control. To let them know, you and I have to establish new priorities. If you resent a family suggestion that your attitudes and behavior are self-defeating ... then they have every right to question the importance of weight control in your life. If we commit ourselves, then we must learn to accept the help our family tries to give. Open communication between partners, family members, and friends will be of utmost importance in lifelong Slim Living.

We must learn how our family or friends can help most effectively in our Slim Life. It certainly does not help, when I take a big bite of ice cream, if a "friend" accuses, "Are you supposed to have that? I caught you again!" That kind of help makes me mad. *No one* should be blamed for obesity. Eating is a learned behavior and there should be neither moral value nor stigma attached to it. There is no blame to fix; we want family support, not censure. My grandma used to say, "You can catch more flies with honey than with vinegar." Confide your day-by-day objectives. If you are attempting to eat only in a seated position at the proper place, ask for a reminder when you forget, but also ask for praise and credit when you accomplish this task. I glow and grow with kind words and praise. I know how "bad" I am . . . we are all filled with enough self-recrimination—we don't need help in that way—but we can never get enough compliments and warm words.

In his book, *Learning to Eat . . . Behavior Modification for Weight Control*, Dr. James N. Ferguson offers some excellent ideas. He suggests:

> Those around you have different styles of reacting to your weight loss. Some patterns of interaction are common, however. Interactions which are painful to the person trying to lose weight should be avoided if they are anticipated and strategies

worked out in advance for coping with them. These interactions do not occur because people are bad, evil or mean, but because people involved are not fully conscious of them or the harmful effect they can have. They are from past habits and they persist because the need has not been there to change.

Some of the most common feelings through the eyes of one trying to lose weight are:

1. No one seems to be interested in what I'm doing or in changing their own habits; others have bad eating habits and do not seem to care.
2. My attempts to change are not supported; they are even ridiculed. Often people say the wrong things. They do not mean to hurt my feelings, but they do.
3. I am discouraged, belittled, made to feel different, and even the butt of jokes. People tease me about my weight even though I am changing and losing.
4. My efforts to change are ignored; my family and friends are always pessimistic, often despite my success.
5. My loss of weight is praised, but when I try to maintain my weight loss and behavior change, they seem to forget and withdraw their support.
6. I feel like I am being sabotaged. It is obvious to me, but I can't do anything about it.
   a. They give me high-calorie treats as presents.
   b. They insist I have high-calorie treats for them or the children.
   c. They continue the pattern ... togetherness is an evening out with a good meal ... we cannot be together without food.

    d. They bring me food at inappropriate
       times (e.g., while I am watching TV).
    e. They use food as a sign of affection;
       it puts me in a bind.
    f. They say I'm becoming too skinny or
      unhealthy.

The reasons for these reactions are numerous. We can only guess about them. Some family members may not want to have to match your self-control, especially if they weigh too much themselves. They may not want things to change. They may be afraid that when you look nicer you will go away, or they won't have anything to complain about. However, the most probable explanation is, that this is the only way they have learned to interact with you when you are losing weight. It is a way that has worked in the past. It is a type of behavior neither one of you has been fully aware of. Fortunately, it is a behavior that is quite amenable to change.

1. Ask for support.
2. Ask for praise. A compliment at the right time will go further than any material reward whether it is money or cream puffs.
3. Ask for feedback and thank them for it.

Remember, many of the behaviors you are changing are hard to detect. Many of your changes are in the form of stopping bad habits, like eating fast, or eating in a different place. People around you will not intuitively know how to compliment you for eating less or not finishing everything on your plate, unless they know your goals. If this program is to succeed, and if you expect to lose weight and maintain that weight loss, then those behaviors must have positive consequences. They have to pay off! You must

100

feel like it has been worth it. If your family and friends have been directly involved in the process of your weight loss, your success is also their success. Your mutual life will be better, and probably longer.

We are grateful to Dr. Ferguson for allowing us to share his ideas with you. Today's assignments incorporate his suggestions, helping you to involve others in your Slim Life. Each day you use one or more of these ideas with someone who cares about you, check in the box marked "Family Involvement."

1. Ask someone for what you want . . . praise, cooperation, feedback, rewards of any kind except food.

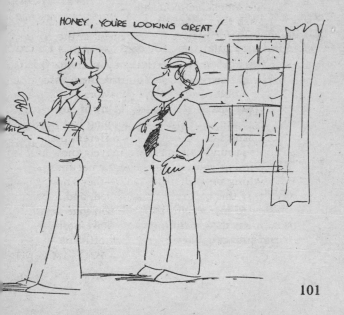

101

2. Tell friends that gifts of food are difficult. You love their thoughtfulness, but a kiss, a flower, or an entertainment trip is preferred.

3. Tell someone close to you specifically what you are trying to accomplish. "Today I will isolate all negative thoughts and evaluate their effects on my food habits. Help me by saying, 'That's negative,' if I forget."

4. Entertain with low-calorie foods. Tell your family you'd appreciate their verbal support.

5. Ask your family to avoid eating problem foods around you . . . ice cream, potato chips, and candy. It's impossible to watch someone else eat and not feel resentful. My young son ate small bags of potato chips outside the house and brushed his teeth before he came close enough for me to smell them.

6. Eliminate foods from your conversation. Recipes, new restaurants, and party plans are strong salient food cues.

7. Find a regular time for exercise with a friend who will work with you. A long walk is more fun when there are two of you. You need exercise, not food.

8. Ask friends not to offer food. It's hard to say "No" when someone insists on sharing. Choose an idea for today and *trust* someone to care enough to help you.

> *A true friend unbosoms freely, advises justly, assists readily, adventures boldly, takes all patiently, defends courageously, and continues a friend unchangeably.*
>
> —WILLIAM PENN

lesson twenty-six

Our Children

"Fatty ... Fatty ... two-by-four
Can't get through the kitchen door."

Remember that childhood musical chant? How often tears are held back as taunts follow the child plagued with overweight. Children can be cruel, but they also speak the truth. A heavy child is fat ... overweight; it cannot be said in a more honest way. Relatives murmur "chubby" or "pleasingly plump," but that doesn't help. They are *different*. Growing up is tough enough, but a tubby endures humiliating experiences which change and warp normal personalities.

Chubby kids are rarely *overactive*. While the thin child playfully wrestles on the floor and laughingly bounces on Daddy's back ... the pudgy runs from competition and finds comfort in a book or TV.

If "baby fat" grows with the child, high school memories may be filled with dateless weekends, oversized clothes, and the solace of pizza, cokes, and French fries. What a shame to miss the wonderful joys of youth because of overweight! Parents can help, if they will face the problem before this introvert has missed the Happy Days of childhood. We, as caring adults, should look at the children around us, our own, our grandchildren, younger brothers and sisters, or perhaps just children whose paths cross ours. How can we help?

1. Show the child we care. Don't nag about food. Give compliments when they are due. Encourage a nice appearance.

2. Take a look at your shape. Ask a child to help you begin to control weight. You could work together, planning meals, packing lunches, fixing snacks. It's fun to help someone else, and children will enjoy helping you.

3. When a child is hurt or sad, never console with foods, saying, "Don't cry, Johnny, have a cookie." Food becomes equated with love in a child's mind, and a "cobweb" habit formed this early soon becomes a strong cablelink to emotions most difficult to break.

4. Encourage any child to participate in physical activities. Better yet, participate with him. Long walks make exciting games. Look for birds, for colors, kick a stone along a sidewalk; children can dream up a million other games. Skating, swimming, and biking encourage a child to develop habits of physical activity. And, incidentally, you will benefit too; it's a two-way advantage!

5. Limit the hours spent in sitting inactively. Start with TV. If we allow hours of TV-sitting each day, our children miss the activity and exercise of

normal, healthful growth. Talk to a child and teach him *how to choose* activities which will be beneficial and fun.

Technique for the day: If there is a child in your life who can use a Slim Living friend, make an effort day by day to help him understand himself, his needs, and your concern. When you do . . . give yourself a check. A little Slender Loving Care may be the best gift you will ever give.

lesson twenty-seven

Future Maintaining

By now I hope you have found some Slim Living ideas and techniques which work for you, your situation, and your personality. Make them a part of your Slim Life-style. Habits deeply ingrained in us are so hard to change. Awareness of new life habits constantly practiced will help you maintain the happiness of being slim.

No one "diet" or style will cover every situation. We are different people at different times, but we need our "heads on straight" at all times. A friend deeply involved in Marriage Enrichment programs offered a tip which seemed applicable to you and me and our food habits. Each morning Pat and her husband spend five minutes together dialoguing about their emotions. If she feels restless and bored with repetitive chores, she lets him know. If he is worried about an office situation, he lets her know. If either is overbusy, they exchange concerns. In this way, they are in tune with each other. Voicing these emotions aloud makes them aware of personal inner emotions. Couldn't we use this technique with our food concerns?

We worry about maintaining weight once it is lost, and rightly so. Failure statistics as high as 80 percent face those who lose ten to forty pounds, whether the diet is self-imposed, directed by a physician, with exercise, or with a supportive class group. Of the 20 percent who succeed in losing and keeping the weight off for a period of six months, less than half maintain the loss permanently. I personally feel you must maintain the loss for a maximum of five years before you feel some degree of security. Even then, you must not neglect the awareness of Living Slim.

Then how do we maintain this loss? Each person must develop his own unique style. In the classes I teach, I help each person discover what foods his or her life-style demands most, which foods are liable to be trouble spots, how to substitute, and how to control amounts of high-calorie foods.

Let me list some of these alternatives, and you decide which might be appropriate for your Slim Life. The trick is, of course, to be aware and alert and to *make* things happen for you instead of *allowing* things to happen *to you*.

1. Some people use an alternating day plan. With this method of maintaining, you stay with your Basic Slim Living plan every other day. On the alternating days you allow yourself one *planned* extra food. For example: Monday I would eat a well-varied basic menu. On Tuesday, I would plan

well in advance to have a small, controlled portion of the high-caloried dessert at my church meeting. At first with this method, it helps to plan each day in advance, whether it be a regular basic food day or a planned, controlled extra-food day. Planning is the key. It eliminates guilt and it allows normal foods, if you still consider high-calorie foods "normal" and low-calorie nutritious foods "abnormal."

2. Others may find the daily extra is possible. It's important to always ask yourself when you decide to enjoy a high-calorie food or an extra-nutritious food, "Do I really want this now or would I prefer something later in the day? If I decide on this food, how much will I eat?" This dialogue with yourself puts *you*, not the food or the situation, in control. This method works well for many.

3. Some are most tempted by problem foods on weekends. The best maintenance technique for them is to stay strictly with the basic plan during the week and allow themselves "controlled extras" on the weekends. It's the amount that makes the difference; there's no kidding your body when you overdo. You and I could eat chocolate ice cream every day of the week and still lose weight, IF . . . we could stop at one level tablespoon each day.

4. Once the weight is down, some find it can be controlled by adding daily exercise. Why not consider group situations such as the YMCA, recreation departments, and adult education classes? Group reinforcement will give you the added incentive of social atmosphere without food involvement. Or, if you prefer a good book, C. Kunzelman's *Activetics* or Clayton Myer's *Official YMCA*

Physical Fitness Handbook will help personalize a program for you.

5. My last suggestion is the most dangerous. Some use calorie-count substitution for maintaining. At this point you realize that weight loss cannot occur over a long period of time simply by your counting calories. If there is a food you crave, it may be better to admit that fact. Figure the calories in a controlled amount and plan them into your daily menu for a day or two, or until that food no longer appeals to you. Care and caution must be used in this conflict of common sense versus emotional uncontrol.

Remember, day by day, you must be aware of your emotions and in control of your responses. If you are ready for maintaining, choose the suggestion which will work best for you and begin . . . today. If you still have a distance to go in the learning cycle . . . wait until the next time around . . . and smile . . .

yet another break

Stop and evaluate. It's time to reflect, where have you been... how are you coming... where are you going? What you begin today is no magical portent for tomorrow. But if you faithfully try, day by day, there will be a tomorrow in your future that brings success, satisfaction, and self-esteem.

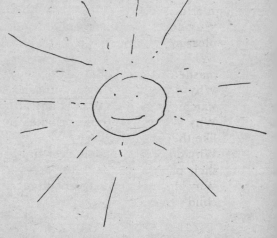

lesson twenty-eight

Random Thoughts

There are days when the martyr complex envelops us, no matter how sensible we try to be. Life's misfortunes happen only to us. At that point, I write down all the nasty things I can think of, and then I laugh at myself.

..... Why do slim women choose friends who are pleasingly plump?

..... Why do church dinners always include mashed potatoes and cake?

..... Why do I always seem hungrier when I'm watching my food than at any other time?

..... Why won't my summer clothes fit this year like they did last year?

..... Why don't thin people ever finish what's on their plates?

..... Why do mothers nag about food left on a child's plate?

..... Why must I "straighten" the cut of pie or cake by nibbling just a little bite?

..... Why does Mother always offer extra-fattening foods when I go home to visit?

..... Why are the most broadening things about travel the little eating places along the way?

..... Why do magazines always show pictures of mouth-watering desserts in delectable color?

..... Why do tempting leftovers in the kitchen have voices of their own, that beg "Eat me ... Eat me"?

..... Why does the favorite menu for any crowd include baked beans, potato salad, ham, and cake?

..... Why can my husband eat twice as much as I and not gain an ounce?

CONCLUSION .....

If I want to control my weight, I must ...

..... Take responsibility for myself and not place the blame on others ...

..... Always be aware of my food intake and calories burned ...

..... Concentrate on keeping records of the foods I consume ...

..... Spend more time in cooking low-calorie foods ...

..... Learn to enjoy myself ... living ... not "DIE-ting."

Here's a test that will help improve your own mental image. In a left-hand column on a piece of paper, write down everything you can think of that makes you mad or unhappy with yourself and your life.

112

Now . . . in a column on the right side, list everything you love about life, about those around you and about yourself. Include at least ten ideas on each list.

Evaluate the importance of each idea. Are the negative things really important or can you live with them? Can they be changed or can you live with them? Can they be changed or are they out of your control? Do the positive thoughts outweigh the negative? When you take the time to analyze pressures and values in your life in this way, give yourself a check in the box marked "Random Thought."

Today my list includes:

Negative
1. My heavy legs.
2. My food cravings.
3. My occasional tardiness.
4. Work pressures I exert on myself.
5. My closets that need cleaning.
6. Never having enough time for everything.
7. Shyness with others.
8. The high cost of everything.
9. The winter weather.
10. Getting up in the morning.

Positive
1. God's love for me.
2. My husband (He's the best!).
3. Good physical and mental health of the children.
4. My new grand-daughter.
5. My boundless energy.
6. Good, warm friends.
7. Personal learned motivation.
8. The seventy pounds lost and kept off.
9. Our home on the river.

10. Every sunny beautiful day.
11. Sound physical health and the desire to keep it.
12. The joy of music.
13. A community and country I love.
14. My good old dog.
15. Vacations in the sun.
16. I almost forgot to stop.

lesson twenty-nine

Which Will It Be?

In the past chapters we have given you ideas to try. If they were appropriate to you and your Slim Life, we hope you accepted them. Remember that all things cannot be learned at one time. If some parts of the ideas we have shared have been useful to you, write them down at the end of this chapter. Review them at least once every four days; see which you are concentrating on during that period.

I believe that many of us with "fat heads" find it difficult to concentrate on any one idea or technique for too long a time. We call it lack of willpower. Willpower is not something God has given to a few and not to others. Willpower is gained through practice, concentration, and awareness. We suggest that after four days you review those ideas which are most helpful to you. Set a goal, for four days only, and work with one or two techniques. At the end of four more days, reevaluate and set another goal. *When we are not working toward a goal . . . we are virtually doing* nothing. . . . Let me repeat . . . *When you are not doing* something . . . *You are doing* nothing.

Don't be misled into thinking weight loss is easy. No one can just sit back and relax while this machine or that method rolls the weight off. Until medical science discovers some conclusive evidence why our systems do not function as others do, we will be responsible for our own losses or gains. There is no easy way, but the rewards in accomplishment are most gratifying.

An unknown poet shares this thought:

> *My body is a house, I build for me,*
> *Myself the architect shall be;*
> *I cannot escape the stubborn fact*
> *That I am fashioned by every act*
> *Which I must determine with my own will,*
> *And there I live, for good or ill.*

To receive your check in the box for Lesson 29, review those ideas which made you aware of reasons for eating and not overeating . . . write down each helpful technique:

_____

_____

_____

_____

_____

_____

In the final analysis, dear friend, the last chapter must be written by YOU . . .

A new Slim Life is not an impossible dream; it's a completely realistic goal. The prescription is simple: You, your desire and determination, plus our helpful techniques are carefully, lovingly mixed. Take them in small, faithful doses. Then treat yourself to the sweet taste of slim living success . . . day by wonderful day.

Day by day, day by day,
Dear Lord, of thee three things I pray:
To see thee more clearly,
Love thee more dearly,
Follow thee more nearly,
Day by day.

—ST. RICHARD OF CHICHESTER

An Appendix of Food Ideas

SUGGESTED DAILY OUTLINE OF BASIC FOODS FOR A SLIM LIFE

BREAKFAST

High vitamin C fruit (see list)

Protein food . . . choose one:

   1 oz. Swiss or Muenster cheese

   1 egg

   1 oz. cooked or canned fish

   2 oz. cottage cheese, farmer, pot, or ricotta

Bread or cereal, whole grain or enriched . . . choose one:

   1 slice bread

   1/2 cup cooked cereal

   3/4 cup ready-to-eat cereal

Coffee or tea if desired

LUNCH

Protein food . . . Choose one:

   2 oz. fish, poultry, or lean meat

   2 oz. Swiss or Muenster cheese

   2 oz. cottage cheese

   1 T. (level) peanut butter

Bread . . . whole grain or enriched . . . 1 slice

Vegetables—Group A . . . three to five choices, raw or cooked—(see list)

Beverage if desired

DINNER

Protein food . . . Choose one:
   3-4 oz. cooked fish, poultry, or lean meat
Vegetables . . . Group A . . . two or more servings
               Group B . . . 1/2 cup cooked or raw
Beverage if desired

OTHER DAILY FOODS

Fats: choose three from list
Milk: 2 cups skimmed or buttermilk or 2/3 cup
       skimmed evaporated
Fruit: three servings from list

FOOD FACTS AND CHOICES

Limit lean beef, pork, and lamb to 12 oz. total
per week
Limit eggs to four per week
Limit hard cheeses to 4 oz. per week
Good low-fat meat choices are fish, chicken
without skin, veal, turkey.

Note: Men could add two extra bread choices per
day and an extra fruit amount.

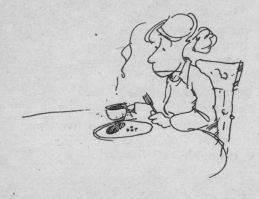

FRUIT CHOICES: No sugar added

Apple, 1 small (2" diam.)

Applesauce, 1/2 cup

Apricots, fresh, 2 med.

Apricots, dried, 4 halves

Banana, 1/2 small

Berries (blackberries, raspberries, *strawberries), 1 cup

Blueberries, 2/3 cup

*Cantaloupe, 1/4 (6" diam.)

Cherries, 10 large

Dates, 2

Figs, fresh, 1 large

Figs, dried, 1 large

*Grapefruit, 1/2 small

*Grapefruit juice, 1/2 cup

Grapes, 12

Grape juice, 1/4 cup

Honeydew melon, 1/8 (7" diam.)

Mango, 1/2 small

*Orange, 1 small

*Orange juice, 1/2 cup

Papaya, 1/3 med.

Peach, 1 med.

Pear, 1 small

Pineapple, 1/2 cup

Pineapple juice, 1/3 cup

Plums, 2 med.

Prunes, dried, 2

Raisins, 2 T.

*Tangerine, 1 large

Watermelon, 1 cup

*These fruits are rich sources of vitamin C; one serving a day should be used.

VEGETABLES:

Group A—You may eat any amount of these vegetables, if they are uncooked. If cooked, a single cupful is permitted.

Asparagus	Chard	*Peppers,
*Broccoli	Collards	green or red
*Brussels	Dandelion	Radishes
sprouts	Kale	Romaine
Cabbage	Mustard	Rhubarb
Cauliflower	Poke	(without
Celery	Spinach	sugar)
*Chicory	Turnip	Sauerkraut
Cucumber	greens	String beans,
Eggplant	Lettuce	young
*Escarole	Mushrooms	Squash,
*Greens	Okra	summer
Beet greens	*Parsley	*Tomatoes
		*Watercress

Group B—One serving equals 1/2 cup.

Beets	Peas, green	*Squash,
*Carrots	Pumpkin	winter
Onions	Rutabagas	Turnips

*These vegetables have a high vitamin A content; at least one serving a day should be used.

FATS: Choose three daily choices
   1 teaspoon vegetable oil
   1 teaspoon mayonnaise
   2 teaspoons French dressing
   1 teaspoon oleo (with liquid vegetable oil listed
      first on label of ingredients)
   1 slice bacon (be careful with weekly amounts)
   6 small nuts

FOODS THAT NEED NOT BE MEASURED:

Coffee	Mustard
Tea	Sweeteners
Clear broth	Pepper, spices
Bouillon (fat free)	Seasonings
Lemon juice	Vinegar
Gelatin (unsweetened)	Sugar-free soft drinks
Rennet tablets	Club soda

Slim Living Recipes

Remember, Living Slim doesn't mean just eating foods from the recipes you find here. I'd rather you begin taking a closer look at the recipes in your own file, in the newspapers and magazines ... creating your own lower-calorie versions of old favorites.

But ... just to give you a start ... try these on for size.

VEGETABLES ...
THE MOST IMPORTANT INGREDIENT

SEVEN WONDER SALAD

2 c. cabbage or 1/2 med. head
1/2 green pepper
1 t. pimiento
1/2 t. chives
1/2 t. parsley or 2 stalks celery
1 T. mushrooms or 3 radishes
1/2 cup French style green beans, drained

Finely chop or grate above ingredients. Mix together in blender, add 1 apple, cored, skin still on, 1/2 cup crushed pineapple, 1/2 t. liquid sweetener, 2 T. white vinegar. Blend until apple is well chopped. Mix salad and fruit mixture together. 1/2 recipe = 1 fruit.

SAUERKRAUT SALAD

1 lrg. can sauerkraut drained and spread out
1/2 c. chopped mushrooms
1/2 c. chopped green pepper
1/2 c. chopped onion
1/2 c. chopped celery
1/2 c. red pepper or pimiento

Layer sauerkraut, mushrooms, green peppers, onions, etc.

SAUCE

1/2 c. wine vinegar
1/4-1/2 c. sweetener
3 t. mustard
2 T. Worcestershire sauce
Kikkoman soy sauce

Put in blender and add salt and pepper; pour over sauerkraut and vegetables, refrigerate 2-3 hrs. (the longer the better).

THREE BEAN SALAD

2 c. or 1 lb. undrained green beans
2 c. or 1 lb. yellow wax beans
2 c. or 1 lb. drained and rinsed bean sprouts
1/2 c. or 1 med. thinly sliced onion
1/4 c. of green pepper or pimiento

1/4 c. of brown Sugar Twin
1 t. celery salt
1/2 t. regular salt
1/2 t. black pepper
3/4 c. cider vinegar
1 t. Worcestershire sauce

In a large mixing bowl, combine all ingredients, cover and chill overnight before serving. Drain well, toss slightly and serve. Leftovers can be stored in refrigerator for several days.

ONIONS ALMONDINE

In saucepan, combine 3/4 c. hot water and one chicken bouillon cube, 1/2 t. almond extract, 1/2 t. salt. Bring to boil. Add 8 oz. peeled and sliced onions. Cover and simmer about 10 minutes or until onions are tender. Recipe = 2 B vegetable servings.

SALAD ARMENIAN

1 cucumber, diced
3 tomatoes, cut in chunks
1/2 c. chopped parsley
1/4 c. chopped mint (or 1/2 t. peppermint extract)
1/2 t. salt
1 t. lemon juice

Toss; chill; count as your sugar vegetable (B).

CASSEROLES

ITALIAN LUNCHEON

Sauce Italiano: In saucepan combine and bring to boil: 8 oz. tomato juice, 1 squirt sweetener, dash salt and any or all of the following: 1/8 t. oregano, 1 small bay leaf, 1 pinch basil, 1 t. onion flakes, dash pepper, 1 t. green pepper chopped, 1 t. celery chopped, mushrooms. When sauce comes to boil, add 1 pkg. frozen cauliflower. Cover and simmer 3-4 minutes. Uncover and boil about 5 minutes till sauce reduced and thick and cauliflower tender. Stir gently to avoid sticking. Reduce heat to simmer. Place Muenster cheese on top of cauliflower. Cover to melt cheese.

BARBECUED TUNA

Cut up celery stalk, 1/2 green pepper, and 1 T. onion flakes. Cover with water and cook till tender, then drain. Add 1/2 c. tomato juice, dash garlic powder, 1 T. soy sauce, 3 oz. tuna fish. Cook till thick. You may add mushrooms.

HOT TUNA SALAD

(You may use chicken or shrimp.)
Mix and place in small Pam-sprayed casserole dish:
2 1/2 oz. tuna
1 big celery stalk, chopped
1 pimiento, chopped

126

1/4 green pepper chopped
1 t. chives
1 t. parsley

Make dressing and pour over top. For dressing:
stir together (don't beat) 1 egg white, 1 T. mayonnaise, 1 to 2 t. lemon juice, 1 squirt sweetener.
Grate 2/3 oz. Swiss cheese on top. Crumble 1 slice
fresh bread in blender and sprinkle on top, too.
Bake at 425° for 15 minutes. Equals 1 fish-cheese
serving, 1 fat, 1 bread, 5 vegetables.

EASY FISH CHOWDER

In saucepan, place 1 cup coarsely chopped carrots,
1 cut up tomato; 3/4 c. onion, chopped; 1/2 c.
celery chopped; 1 bay leaf; 1 chopped green pepper; pepper; 1 t. chopped parsley. Bring to boil
and simmer 15 minutes (other vegs. may be
added). Add 1 12 oz. package thawed fillet of cod.
Simmer 15 minutes more until fish flakes easily
with fork. Remove solids and let broth boil until
there is only about 1 cup left. Flake fish and return
all to chowder. Stir in 1/3 cup powdered milk and
heat.

ORIENTAL SALAD

1 can bean sprouts
1 small can mushroom pieces
1 large stalk finely chopped celery
1 finely diced pimiento
1/8 t. instant minced garlic
liquid from mushrooms
salt and pepper to taste
water
1/2 c. vinegar
1 t. liquid sweetener
1/4 t. each ginger and cinnamon
1/8 t. each turmeric, clove, and nutmeg
1 T. soy sauce

Drain and rinse bean sprouts. Drain mushrooms, and cook celery 15 minutes in the liquid. Drain celery and measure liquid, adding sufficient water to give 1/2 cups altogether. Combine all vegetables. Also mix all other ingredients, except salt and pepper, in a saucepan, and bring to a boil. Pour over vegetable combination, season with salt and pepper, and chill before serving.

TOMATO CASSEROLE

2 c. cooked tomatoes
1 lg. onion, diced
1 green pepper, diced
1 red pepper, diced
3 stks. celery, small chunks
1 t. salt

Cook until celery is tender. Spray bowl with Pam. Add vegetables. Sprinkle with 3 oz. Swiss cheese diced. Bake 1 hour at 350°.

RED CABBAGE WITH APPLE

2 to 3 c. shredded red cabbage
4 oz. chopped onion
1 tart apple, peeled, cored, and diced
Sweetener to equal 1 T. sugar. Salt to taste.
1/4 c. vinegar, 1/4 t. caraway seed.

Combine apple, onion, and cabbage in a saucepan and barely cover with water. Cover and simmer 30 minutes. Uncover and add sweetener and salt. If most of water is not gone, increase heat until it is. Add vinegar and caraway seed. Stir well and heat through.

FRIED CABBAGE

Cabbage (shredded)
Salt and black pepper
Sweetener
Vinegar

Fry cabbage in Pam-coated fry pan on low heat, stirring often. When cabbage is slightly brown, season lightly with salt and pepper. When nice and brown (just before you take off heat) add vinegar and sweetener to taste, mixing thoroughly.

FRUIT AND VEGETABLE SLAW
WITH SWEET-SOUR DRESSING

Dressing: 2/3 c. orange juice
2 T. Lemon juice, 1 T. brown sugar substitute
1 egg, beaten
1/2 t. salt, 1/2 t. basil
1/2 t. mint
Slaw: 1 head iceburg lettuce, shredded
1 large apple, coarsely grated, 2 medium carrots,
1 cucumber, chopped.

For dressing, combine orange juice, lemon juice, brown sugar, egg, salt, basil, and mint in top of double boiler. Set over boiling water and cook, stirring constantly until slightly thickened. Cool. For slaw; core, rinse, and thoroughly drain lettuce. Shred lettuce and turn into salad bowl. Arrange apple, carrot, and cucumber on top. Pour sweet-sour dressing over and toss slightly to blend. Makes 6 servings.

WALDORF SALAD

Dice 3 medium apples. Drizzle 1 t. lemon juice over them to keep the color. Mix 2 1/2 cups thin celery strips, about 1 inch long; 12 diced walnut halves; sweetener to equal 1 T. sugar (if desired); and 1/2 cup low-fat yogurt. Stir well, chill, and serve on lettuce leaves. Whole recipe is 3 fruit, 2 fat, and 1/2 milk.

PEANUT BUTTER LUNCHEON TREATS

Combine: 2/3 cup dry milk, 1/2 cup oatmeal,
2 T. peanut butter; 1 t. vanilla;
1/2 t. cinnamon; 1 cup lo-cal applesauce.
Sweeten to taste.

Bake at 350° for 15-20 minutes. 1/2 recipe equals
1 milk, 1 fruit, 1 protein, 1 bread.

ORIENTAL SKILLET

Brown 8 oz. ground beef, veal, or tuna with 1
onion chopped. Add 1 large can chop suey vegetables, 1 can drained mushrooms, 1/4 t. ginger,
3 T. soy sauce, sweetener to equal 1 t. sugar.
Simmer. 1/2 recipe is a dinner protein.

CHEESE DELIGHT

1 slice bread (broken in pieces)
1/4 t. onion powder; 1/2 c. chopped pepper;
1 4-oz can mushrooms, salt and pepper to taste;
2 oz. hard cheese (Swiss or Muenster)
Save 1/2 oz. cheese; 1/2 c. tomato juice

Mix all ingredients and place in a casserole dish.
Grate reserved 1/2 oz. cheese over the top. Bake at
350° for 1 1/2 hours.

RAISIN BREAD PUDDING

In baking dish, combine 1 cup skim milk; 1 slice bread cut in cubes; 1 egg beaten (or the equivalent of Egg Beaters); 1/2 t. vanilla; 1/4 t. cinnamon; 1/4 t. nutmeg; sweetener to equal 1/2 cup sugar; 1 T. raisins. Set in pan of water about 1" deep. Bake at 375° — 40 minutes till set.

PINEAPPLE UPSIDE-DOWN CAKE

8 slices pineapple
1 c. pineapple juice
3 t. sweetener
1 t. cinnamon
1 t. vanilla
1 t. coconut flavoring

Simmer 10 minutes. Set aside 1 1/3 cup dry skim milk; 2 t. sweetener; pinch cinnamon; 2 pkgs. gelatin; 1/2 cup cold water; 1/2 cup hot water. Pour over pineapple mixture. Place in 9 " pie tin. Sprinkle milk mixture over filling. Sprinkle with water on top. Press with spoon. Bake 350° for 20 minutes. 1/2 pie = 2 milk, 2 fruits.

CHOCOLATE BANANA CUPCAKES

2/3 c. chocolate Alba dry milk
2 eggs; banana; 1/2 t. baking soda;

1/2 t. vanilla; 1/2 t. cream tartar;
1 slice bread, crumbled

Blend about 7 minutes till liquid. Fill cupcake tins.
Bake 325° for 25 minutes. 3 cupcakes = breakfast.
Recipe makes 6.

FRUIT MUFFINS

1 apple or 1 banana or 1 c. applesauce
2/3 c. dry milk
2 eggs
1/4 t. salt
5 T. cornmeal or oatmeal
1 T. sweetener or less
1 t. walnut or butter pecan extract
1/4 t. baking powder.

Mix together. Bake in muffin tin at 350° for 20
minutes. 1/2 = 1 fruit, 1 milk, and 1/2 bread, 1 egg.

PINEAPPLE CRISP

1/2 c. pineapple chunks (packed in own juice) or
1/2 small fresh pineapple cubed
1/3 c. powdered milk
1/4 c. water

Mix 1/2 of milk and 1/2 of water and pineapple
in small baking dish. Sprinkle with cinnamon,
sweetener, and rest of milk powder. Cover and
bake at 350° for 25 minutes or until tender.

CRANBERRY WHIP

1 1/2 c. cranberries
3/4 c. boiling water
sweetener to taste
3 egg whites
1 t. grated orange rind
1 t. lemon juice

Cook cranberries in water until skins burst (about 5 minutes). Cool. Put through blender. Add sweetener. Beat egg whites until stiff. Add cranberries, orange rind, and lemon juice. Beat until glossy and stiff. Chill.

FRUIT DELIGHT

1/2 lb. cottage cheese
1 tangerine
1 banana
1 apple
1 pkg. Knox gelatine
sweetener to taste

Put all ingredients in blender until smooth. Refrigerate until set. Garnish with bananas, tangerine sections, and allspice. Breakfast or lunch. 1/2 recipe = 1/2 c. cottage cheese and 2 fruits.

FROZEN CUSTARD

While blender is running, add 4 oz. pop (any flavor) or boiling water; 1 pkg. gelatin; 1/3 cup powdered milk; or 1/2 t. fruit extract to conform with flavor used; 1/2 t. vanilla.

Add 4-6 ice cubes (one at a time) until custard consistency is reached.

PEPPERMINT BAVARIAN

1 packet unflavored gelatin
1/4 c. cold water
1 1/2 c. skim milk liquid
3 drops artificial sweetener
1/4 t. peppermint extract
4 drops red food coloring
1/3 c. Alba skim milk powder

Soften gelatin in cold water. Heat 1 1/2 cup milk and sweetener, stirring constantly, until bubbles form around edges of pan. Add gelatin, add extract, coloring; chill until slightly thickened. Pour 1/3 cup water into 1-quart bowl. Sprinkle 1/3 cup dry milk over surface and beat until stiff. Fold into gelatin mixture and spoon lightly into sherbet glasses.

LUNCHEON DELIGHT

1 pkg. cherry D-Zerta
8 oz. cottage cheese
2 pears
1/4 t. almond extract

Prepare D-Zerta as directed on box. Blend cottage cheese and pears until smooth. Add extract. Divide D-Zerta in half, add cheese-pear mixture to half, use other to garnish. Mold. Chill. 1/2 = 4 oz. cheese and 1 fruit.

LIME COTTAGE CHEESE MOLD

2 envelopes lime D-Zerta
2 c. boiling water
1 can crushed pineapple
1 16 oz. carton cottage cheese

Dissolve gelatin thoroughly in hot water. Stir in pineapple and cottage cheese. Chill and serve cold. Display mold on lettuce.

PIPPIN' DIET REDPOP APPLE SALAD

1 3/4 c. diet red cream soda
1 T. lemon juice
1/2 c. water
1 can (16 oz.) diet applesauce
2 envelopes unflavored gelatin
red food coloring
1/4 t. cinnamon
whole cloves

Heat diet red cream soda over low heat but do not boil. Sprinkle gelatin over water and allow to soften. Stir into soda with cinnamon, lemon juice, and applesauce and stir until gelatin is dissolved. Add red food coloring if desired for a deeper color. Cool slightly, then pour into well-oiled individual custard cups and chill 4-6 hours. Unmold on well-dried lettuce leaves. Insert whole cloves in the top of each to resemble apple stem and garnish with 2 or 3 mint leaves if desired. Serves 6 to 8. Serve with low-calorie topping if desired.

PEAR ALMONDINE

1 pkg. unflavored gelatin
1/4 t. almond extract
4-6 t. sweetener
1/4 c. cold water
1/4 c. boiling water
2/3 c. dry milk
1 pear
4-6 ice cubes

Sprinkle gelatin in cold water in blender to soften. Add boiling water, 3/4 of unpeeled pear, cut in small pieces, extract, water, milk, and sweetener. Run at medium speed until mixture is smooth. Add ice cubes one at a time. Run at medium speed after each ice cube till well mixed. Chop remaining pear in small pieces and fold into mixture. Eat immediately. All = 2 milks and 2 fruit.

SEAFOAM SALAD

Chill 1 can evaporated skim milk until very cold. Place 2 cups unsweetened applesauce in saucepan. Sprinkle with 1 pkg. D-Zerta gelatin and heat and stir until gelatin is dissolved. Set aside. Beat milk in a large bowl until soft peaks form. Fold in applesauce and chill. 1/4 recipe = 1 fruit, 3 oz. of skim evaporated milk.

THREE FRUIT SHERBET

1 med. banana
1 16-oz. can crushed pineapple
1/2 of 6-oz. can frozen orange juice
1/2 c. dry milk powder

Blend 30 seconds and freeze.

PUMPKIN COOKIES

4 oz. pumpkin
3 t. sweetener
1 t. cinnamon
1/4 t. ginger
1/2 t. maple flavoring
1/3 c. dry milk

Mix and drop dough on Teflon or Pam-sprayed pan. Bake at 450° for 25 minutes. Tastes like gingerbread.

APPLE-NUT COOKIES

1 medium apple, peeled, cored, and grated
Sweetener to taste
2/3 c. dry skim milk powder
1/2 tsp. cinnamon
dash each of nutmeg and ginger
1/8 t. vanilla
1/4 t. butter pecan flavor

Combine and drop on sprayed cookie sheet. *Bake on top shelf of oven* for 15 minutes at 350°. Equals 2 (8 oz.) servings milk and 1 serving fruit.

APPLESAUCE COOKIES

1 c. unsweetened applesauce
24 nuts
1 1/3 c. dry milk
1/4 c. raisins
1 t. vanilla
1/2 t. cinnamon
sweetener to taste

Mix: applesauce, milk, vanilla, cinnamon, sweetener; add: nuts and raisins. Bake 375° for 10-15 minutes. 1/4 recipe = 1 milk, 1 fruit, 1 fat.

PINEAPPLE COOKIES

Mix 1 cup well-drained crushed pineapple, 1 1/3 cup dry milk powder; 1/2 t. vanilla; sweetener to taste; 1 t. raisins; 6 walnut halves.

Drop by teaspoonfuls on Teflon cookie sheet. Bake 350° for 15-20 minutes.

LICORICE DROPS

5 envelopes Knox gelatin
2-3 t. lime or cherry gelatin
sweetener to taste
3-4 c. boiling water
anise *or* peppermint extract to taste
red *or* green food coloring

Add boiling water to gelatin and stir, cool, and add extract choice, set in refrigerator, cut into squares.

139

MARSHMALLOWS

4 packets unflavored gelatin
1 c. powdered milk
1 c. lo-cal diet cream soda
1/2 t. vanilla
2 drops butter flavoring
1 t. orange extract
16 packs artificial sweetener

Stir gelatin into soda, add milk and beat. Place over low heat just long enough to dissolve gelatin. Add flavoring and gradually add sweetener. Beat until very thick. Pour into pan and chill. When cool, cut into squares.

FINGER JELLO

6 packets unflavored gelatin
2 1/2 T. sweetener
3 Kool-aid (any flavor)
2 T. lemon juice
4 c. water (1 cold, 3 hot)

Dissolve gelatin in cold—heat to dissolve, then add rest of water and other ingredients. Mold in cake pan—cut into small squares.

CHOCOLATE-COCONUT FINGERS

1 can cream soda
sweetener to taste
1/3 c. powdered milk
3 t. chocolate extract

2 t. coconut extract
4 envelopes Knox gelatin

Dissolve gelatin by heating in 1/2 c. of pop. Mix all ingredients. Pour into pan and let set. Recipe = 1 milk.

BEVERAGES

HOT TODDY TEA

1 tsp. orange peel
dash cinnamon
2 whole cloves
4 drops Sweeta
1 tea bag
2 c. boiling water

Steep 5 minutes with all ingredients but sweetener. Serve hot.

"IT-SURE-DOESN'T-TASTE-LIKE-IT"

Mix 4 oz. tomato juice, 4 oz. buttermilk, 1/2 tsp. celery salt, dash onion powder, fresh ground pepper. Serve over 2 ice cubes.

HOT BUTTERED RUM COFFEE

To 4 c. boiling water, add 12 t. instant coffee, 2 tsp. rum extract, 8 whole cloves, 1/2 t. imitation butter flavoring, 6 drops Sweeta, 1/2 c. evaporated skimmed milk. Heat and serve in four cups garnished with cinnamon sticks.

FROSTY ORANGE JELLO

In blender combine 4 ozs. orange juice, 2/3 c. dry milk powder, 8 drops Sweeta, and 15 ice cubes one at a time through top. Blend until crushed. Serves two and equals 1/2 fruit and 1 milk each.

ORANGE-PINEAPPLE PUNCH

Use 1 large can of frozen orange-pineapple juice. Add amount of water listed on can; add sweetener to taste, and 2 qts. low-calorie ginger ale. Combine. Chill. Pour over ice in large punch bowl. Garnish with orange or lime slices.

"COLD DUCK"

Combine 2 bottles diet black cherry pop; 1 can Fresca; 1/4 cup wine vinegar.

HAWAIIAN PUNCH

3 c. unsweetened pineapple juice
2 t. liquid sweetener
1 1/2 c. unsweetened orange juice
2 qts. carbonated water, chilled
3/4 c. unsweetened lemon juice

Combine juices and sweetener. Chill. Just before serving, add carbonated water. If desired, garnish with ice ring or mold. Serve immediately.

BANANA NOG

1 ripe medium banana
1 c. skim milk

1 t. sweetener
1/4 t. nutmeg

Put all ingredients except nutmeg in blender with 1 cup ice cubes and whirl 30 seconds. Pour into tall glasses, dust with nutmeg, and serve at once. Makes 2 glasses.

TOMATO SURPRISE

Combine 6 oz. tomato juice; dash of Worcestershire sauce; dash of pepper.

SAUERKRAUT JUICE COCKTAIL

1 T. lemon juice
1/8 t. caraway seeds
4 oz. sauerkraut juice

Combine lemon juice and caraway seeds in glass. Add ice cubes, then sauerkraut juice. Stir well.

TEA COOLER

1 1/3 c. boiling water
1/2 c. unsweetened orange juice
4 tea bags
1/2 c. unsweetened lemon juice
1 c. unsweetened pineapple juice
1 T. liquid sweetener
1/2 c. unsweetened grapefruit juice
2 c. low-calorie ginger ale.

Pour boiling water over tea bags. Let steep 2 to 3 minutes. Remove tea bags. Add juices and sweetener. Cool. Just before serving, add ginger ale and ice cubes.

acknowledgments

Frank Konishi, *Exercise Equivalents of Foods* (Carbondale: Southern Illinois University Press, 1973).

Charles Kuntzleman, *Activetics* (New York: Peter H. Wyden, 1975).

Jo Carr and Imogene Sorley, *Bless This Mess & Other Prayers* (Nashville: Abingdon Press, 1969, p. 78).

Helen Steiner Rice, "On Wings of Prayer" (Old Tappan, N.J.: Fleming H. Revell Co.).

Jo Carr and Imogene Sorley, *Too Busy Not to Pray* (Nashville: Abingdon Press, 1966).

James N. Ferguson, *Learning to Eat, Behavior Modification for Weight Control* (Palo Alto: Bull Publishing Co., 1975).

Clayton Myers, *The Official YMCA Physical Fitness Handbook*, (New York: Popular Library, 1975).

charts

DAY BY DAY . . . . . FOR A SLIM LIFE

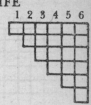

1. Food Inventory
2. Set Your Goal
3. A Work Task Accomplished
4. Analyze Feelings
5. Eating Ratio
6. Plan a Day
7. Weigh Your Meats
8. Take a Walk
9. Increase Caloric Output
10. Slow Down Techniques
11. Further Food Techniques
12. Reduce Overeating Events
13. Eliminate a Negative Thought
14. Relax
15. Evaluation of Appearance and Attitude
16. Cook a Dish
17. Four Glasses of Water
18. Reduce Sugar Consumption (Cold Turkey)
19. A Vegetable Idea
20. The Nutrition Game
21. Plan One Food Event a Day
22. Plan Time
23. Record Points and Awards
24. The Good Deeds Jar
25. Involve Your Family
26. Include a Child
27. Am I Ready to Maintain?
28. Random Thoughts
29. It's Up to You!!

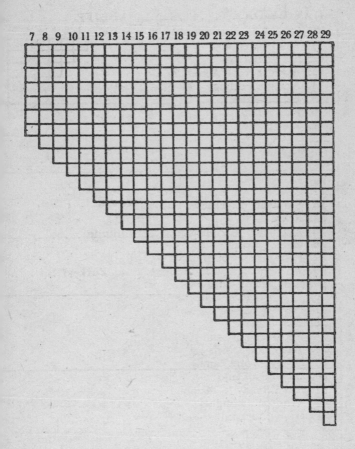

FOOD INTAKE INVENTORY FORM   DAY   NAME

FOOD: AMOUNT	FOOD INVENTORY LIST	TIME OF DAY AND LENGTH OF TIME	SOCIAL DEGREE OF HUNGER (0-4)		PLACE: HOME, WORK RESTAURANT RECREATION	MOOD: ANXIOUS BORED TIRED DEPRESSED ANGRY HAPPY	1. OTHER ACTIVITY 2. BODY POSITION
			ALONE	WITH:			

148

FOOD INTAKE INVENTORY FORM

DAY   NAME

FOOD: AMOUNT	FOOD INVENTORY LIST	TIME OF DAY AND LENGTH OF TIME	SOCIAL — DEGREE OF HUNGER (0-4)		PLACE: HOME, WORK RESTAURANT RECREATION	MOOD: ANXIOUS BORED TIRED DEPRESSED ANGRY HAPPY	1. OTHER ACTIVITY 2. BODY POSITION
			ALONE	WITH:			

FOOD INTAKE INVENTORY FORM   DAY   NAME

FOOD: AMOUNT	FOOD INVENTORY LIST	TIME OF DAY AND LENGTH OF TIME	SOCIAL DEGREE OF HUNGER (0-4)		PLACE: HOME, WORK RESTAURANT RECREATION	MOOD: ANXIOUS BORED TIRED DEPRESSED ANGRY HAPPY	1. OTHER ACTIVITY 2. BODY POSITION
			ALONE	WITH:			

150

FOOD INTAKE INVENTORY FORM

DAY   NAME

FOOD: AMOUNT	FOOD INVENTORY LIST	TIME OF DAY AND LENGTH OF TIME	SOCIAL DEGREE OF HUNGER (0-4)		PLACE: HOME, WORK RESTAURANT RECREATION	MOOD: ANXIOUS BORED TIRED DEPRESSED ANGRY HAPPY	1. OTHER ACTIVITY 2. BODY POSITION
			ALONE	WITH:			

FOOD INTAKE INVENTORY FORM   DAY   NAME

FOOD: AMOUNT	FOOD INVENTORY LIST	TIME OF DAY AND LENGTH OF TIME	SOCIAL		PLACE: HOME, WORK RESTAURANT RECREATION	MOOD: ANXIOUS BORED TIRED DEPRESSED ANGRY HAPPY	1. OTHER ACTIVITY 2. BODY POSITION
			DEGREE OF HUNGER (0-4)				
			ALONE	WITH:			

FOOD INTAKE INVENTORY FORM

DAY _____ NAME _____

FOOD: AMOUNT FOOD INVENTORY LIST	TIME OF DAY AND LENGTH OF TIME	SOCIAL DEGREE OF HUNGER (0-4) / ALONE / WITH:	PLACE: HOME, WORK RESTAURANT RECREATION	MOOD: ANXIOUS BORED TIRED DEPRESSED ANGRY HAPPY	1. OTHER ACTIVITY 2. BODY POSITION

153

FOOD INTAKE INVENTORY FORM DAY NAME

FOOD: AMOUNT	FOOD INVENTORY LIST	TIME OF DAY AND LENGTH OF TIME	SOCIAL DEGREE OF HUNGER (0-4)		PLACE: HOME, WORK RESTAURANT RECREATION	MOOD: ANXIOUS BORED TIRED DEPRESSED ANGRY HAPPY	1. OTHER ACTIVITY 2. BODY POSITION
			ALONE	WITH:			

THINK THIN
for SLIM LIVING

Name _____ Wk. of _____
Wt. _____ Loss _____
Write it down . . . . . You'll Win . . . . . When you Lose

	Mon.	Tues.	Wed.	Thurs.	Fri.	Sat.	Sun.
BREAKFAST							
LUNCH							
DINNER							
Milk							
Fruit							
Beef							
Fish							

THINK THIN
for SLIM LIVING

Name_____ Wk. of _____
Wt._____ Loss_____
Write it down . . . . . You'll Win . . . . . When you Lose

	Mon.	Tues.	Wed.	Thurs.	Fri.	Sat.	Sun.
BREAKFAST							
LUNCH							
DINNER							
Milk							
Fruit							
Beef							
Fish							

THINK THIN
for SLIM LIVING

Name _____ Wk. of _____
Wt. _____ Loss _____
Write it down . . . . . You'll Win . . . . . When you Lose

	Mon.	Tues.	Wed.	Thurs.	Fri.	Sat.	Sun.
BREAKFAST							
LUNCH							
DINNER							
Milk							
Fruit							
Beef							
Fish							

157

THINK THIN
for SLIM LIVING

Name _____ Wk. of _____
Wt. _____ Loss _____
Write it down ..... You'll Win ..... When you Lose

	Mon.	Tues.	Wed.	Thurs.	Fri.	Sat.	Sun.
BREAKFAST							
LUNCH							
DINNER							
Milk							
Fruit							
Beef							
Fish							

THINK THIN
for SLIM LIVING

Name _____ Wk. of _____

Wt. _____ Loss _____

Write it down . . . . . You'll Win . . . . . When you Lose

	Mon.	Tues.	Wed.	Thurs.	Fri.	Sat.	Sun.
BREAKFAST							
LUNCH							
DINNER							
Milk							
Fruit							
Beef							
Fish							